Entry-Level Cancer

My First Six Months in the Club That No One Wants to Join

David Baskett

*For Carina and Kaily
And Cancer-Club members everywhere*

CONTENTS

Thank you Laurie Fox for believing in me, and helping to make this book happen (even though publishers wouldn't touch it because I'm not "somebody"). Thanks Patrick Miller for whittling out words and pages, smoothing flow, and other feats of high-end editing.

Thank you Lance Armstrong, for trying and lying. This sounds sarcastic, but without your post-cancer, Tour de France "wins," Livestrong wouldn't have carried the weight it did (does?). Upon your downfall, I was pissed off and disillusioned. Time passes. You admittedly trained like a wild man and were driven, which inspired and helped me. That's why I left my hero-worship bits in the book (as you will see, I fully believed your story at the time). Let he or she, the un-tainted, regret-free cancer survivor, cast the first stone....

PROLOGUE

Usually it's fun to start a new hobby. But this time I chose basaloid squamous-cell carcinoma, metastatic. Actually it chose me; I would have chosen the piano.

It is nearly Christmas. I read the newspaper, come across the obituaries, and see my face. *I am them.* I am a 72-year-old black woman from La Porte, Texas. I am a blonde cheerleader from Tomball, and a Hispanic baby, still-born in Katy. I am an elderly Vietnamese man and a more elderly white farmer; I look very old in both of those pictures. I am one of three World War II veterans, the one pictured in my prime (I like the sailor hat). There can be any cause of death, at any age; it doesn't matter. I wait. It's only a matter of time.

There are no test results because it is nearly Christmas. Cancer takes a holiday. Actually, quantification takes a holiday; the cancer keeps on keeping on. I do not need results that tell me whether I have cancer, because I *know* that I have cancer. That fact has been established. What I'm waiting for are results that tell me *how much* cancer. In how many nooks and crannies and organs does it reside? Already I suspect that it's everywhere, like Bermuda grass in the garden—it has runners and roots and cannot be stopped. It spreads and takes hold, entangles organs and grows when nobody is looking. I feel it, or I think I do. What is this pain in my side? My pancreas? Lower left of the abdominal cavity; that could be my pancreas. I should look up where a pancreas is supposed to be, when it is not running away from cancer.

In the meantime, the known cancerous lymph node has spewed its spore to places unknown throughout my body, and its offspring have taken root, suckling pigs on the teats of my well-maintained circulatory system—oh, the irony of that—awaiting the moment to come ripping out of my chest at Christmas dinner, then attaching itself to somebody's mouth, only to be killed later by Sigourney Weaver.

I think about death; I ponder it. I must ponder death, because I do not know if that's how this will end. Habit compels me to consider the worst case, for I am an engineer. When in doubt, when crucial information is lacking, one designs for the worst possible case. So I must design my exit strategy, because I might die. No, I *will* die, but I just don't know when.

But as an engineer, I also know that it's possible to err toward the pessimistic. In deference to engineering dogma, I must acknowledge such a possibility. In order to clear up uncertainty and narrow the range of possibilities, I Google my diagnosis.

Minutes pass. Now I *really* know that I'm going to die soon. If it's on the internet it must be true, right?

Or is it?

1 HOW'S LIFE?

In July 2007, I am the healthiest individual I know. During any given week, I work out in the weight room twice, attend two yoga classes and three Taekwondo classes. I am a first-degree black belt; I can kick people in the head, but only after I'm good and warmed up (provided that they don't kick me in the head first, nose in particular). I eat fairly well, with a decent smattering of veggies, although I am not overly fond of the green ones if they've only been steamed. Cheese helps. I sleep enough. I have not had so much as a cold in years. I will step out on a limb and declare myself a freakish anomaly of an American citizen over the age of forty, for I am not overweight, my blood pressure is ideal, my resting heart rate hovers around one beat per second, I do not have Type II diabetes, and I take no prescription medicines.

I have a lovely family. My beautiful wife Jenelle—even her name is lovely—works as an engineer in the oil business. Our eldest daughter Carina, also beautiful, is a sophomore biology major, living on campus at Rice University. Rice is an eclectic oak-tree-filled oasis of academia, born of Houston's desire to legitimize itself as an actual city (still a work in progress). While smart people in Texas are looked upon with suspicion by the natives, Carina rebels. She is in the right place, because Rice is a known safe haven for nerds.

Our youngest daughter Kaily, beauty just blooming, is a bubbly high school freshman who can make me laugh while kicking me in the head, even *before* she is good and warmed up (taekwondo is the family sport). She dances for the joy of it and dreams of flying on the pure strength of her desire, like a proper superhero.

Both girls are ex-gymnasts, well-read, articulate, loving, and fun to be around. As if all that is not enough, we have a yellow Lab named Bonehead, though for some reason the girls insist on calling her Sadie. If Norman Rockwell were alive today and painting suburbanites in Houston, people would see us on the cover of *Life* magazine and say "Norm's losing it, I mean, where's the realism? The dysfunction?"

In my cocoon of loveliness, I try to maintain a low level of stress. I run my own business, and I am the sole employee. Other employees would create stress, and I am big on stress mitigation; for example, I refuse to drive in rush-hour traffic. I make a lot of money, all things being relative—I am an engineer, after all—and try to live in a state of flow. I write fiction at dawn, take morning breaks to sit by the pool and soak up splendors of nature through the filter of a backyard tropical garden (lots of banana trees); then, in the afternoons I invent specialized pieces of equipment for Houston's vast industrial base. I am a renaissance man, age forty-three. I have a lump.

Discovery

Although summer afternoons in Houston can be absurdly uncomfortable, bordering on cruelty ("It's not the heat, it's the humidity!"), I still consider this the best season of the year. Reasons include swimming, long days, lush greenery, and some hammock time now and then. Between hammock visits, snacks, and naps, I pursue the business by strolling to the home office to sit at the computer.

While at the keyboard, I notice now and again an odd numbness down the back of my left arm, and an occasional slight ache in the armpit on the same side. These sensations are unusual, but I chalk them up to overuse or minor freak injuries (I get a lot of those), and file these thoughts away for later consideration. I keep on keeping on, and do not even think of mentioning anything about my slight misgivings to Jenelle. Weeks pass.

On the morning of discovery, I sit alone in the house. I read the newspaper in the sun-drenched breakfast room and drink coffee. The coffee is good; life is good. I gaze out across the swimming pool, a serene and sky-blue pond like the pools one finds in brochures for island destinations, because as a swimming hole an ocean won't suffice, what with its oddly shaped shores and fish poop. There are no meetings planned today; I need not dress beyond a pair of shorts, tee-shirt optional. I decide that I will be wearing the shirt and flip flops when I saunter into the local gym later. I am the king of my world.

The thing is, life hasn't always been this way. I have only recently arrived at this lovely plateau after two soul-killing decades of drowning in the banalities of corporate America. The routine involved maximum stress while fighting the system, followed by lots of drinking, various outbursts of anger and frustration, and corresponding rocky times with Jenelle. Looking back, I'm surprised we've made it this long... but right now, things are much better.

I worked myself up the ladder during the years after college running on pure type-A personality: too much caffeine, aggressive driving, sarcastic quips in every direction. But I have found a small oasis of peace by managing my own firm. Jenelle and I fight less. I have decided that if I can't change, and Lord knows I've tried, then maybe switching career paths can smooth things over. And it seems to be working: I finally feel hopeful about achieving real serenity after all these years.

Banana leaves rustle, bow, then stand tall. I gaze back at the paper, then hear a voice. Not a neighbor or a radio, but a voice in my head saying: *"Check..."* A moment later, it adds, *"...arm."* The message is Tarzan-like, dumb but instinctive. By age forty-three I have learned to listen to my little Tarzan, he-man of my inner jungle. Like reaching for a vine, I extend my left arm skyward. I check around the back of the shoulder, then the triceps, which are numb at this moment. I move my hand under my armpit and probe around, because there's a slight ache in that region.

Probe, nothing. Probe, nothing; sigh with relief and gaze upon the pool. Tarzan keeps grunting. Probe, *something*... I freeze.

What was *that*? I probe again and find nothing, cannot find the *something* that was there for a moment. Then I do: It is a lump. But this must be normal armpit anatomy. I mean, what do I know? I'm not a professional armpit prober. So I feel the right side, confident that I will find a similar lump—ergo, normal anatomy—and then I shall resume coffee drinking and pool-gazing.

But there is no lump on the right side.

Left, right, left, right. Right, no lump. Left, a lump. I have a lump! *A freaking lump!*

The lump—I'll name him Lumpy—is about the size of a mid-grade blueberry. Lumpy is hard, a *frozen* blueberry. I have a frigging frozen blueberry named Lumpy in my left armpit. With the discovery of Lumpy comes a wave of nausea. I want a doctor. *I want a doctor right now!* That's because lumps mean cancer and by the summer of 2007, I already know the outcome of the cancer game: The game is fixed and the house wins. My father-in-law, Jim, played this game a few years back, and he died. The big C equals the big D. Lumpy is a personal friend of the Grim Reaper. I phone my doctor.

Jim died from small-cell lung cancer. He and his wife Jo lived in our house during his treatment at MD Anderson in Houston. MD Anderson is Oz, the Emerald City, the house that cancer built. It is colossal; it would be the Home Depot of cancer treatment except that Home Depot has cement floors and the occasional bargain, and doesn't charge fifteen dollars a day for its patrons to park.

Over the course of two years, we all watched Jim change from a weekly golfer to an increasingly weak oxygen bottle-user. He began as a large man and became a slim one—in a word, gaunt. The house won; he died, neither a good death nor a pretty one. Jenelle and Jo and the girls were destroyed. I tried to be strong for them all, but I cried. He and I had golfed together and yelled at the TV together whenever the Cowboys played. We shared bottles of Scotch; I loved to sit and chill out while he played jazz piano. Then cancer killed him and he was gone.

Thus I know first-hand that people with cancer die, and they do not die good deaths. They die expensive deaths requiring frequent long commutes and tortuous treatments. They become more and more gaunt and then they are gone. Proper engineering dogma does not allow extrapolation based on a single data point, but I ignore all this, extrapolate away, and conclude with a prognosis for all humans diagnosed with cancer: they die. I have a lump, people with lumps have cancer, people with cancer die.

The doctor's receptionist answers the phone. Can you wait until next Tuesday? No? Please don't use that language, sir, I'm only the receptionist. How about a physician's assistant at 2:00 this afternoon? Fine.

Live Strong

Actually, not everyone who gets cancer dies from cancer. There were 1.4-million *new* cases of good old American cancer in 2007. That's a heap of cancer, my friends. So lots of people have it and they're walking around all over the place, living as survivors with fulfilling lives. Lots of them don't talk about it with non-members, but if you get cancer, you're in the club. Club members will talk to you because you're one of *us*. You've been through the wringer; you can understand.

How does one tell if a person is in the club? Are all club members financially strapped, gaunt, or bald, or on death's door? I'm not (yet). Well, I am getting to be a bit bald on top (that's a solar panel for a cancer-surviving machine!).

Cancer patients are essentially a survival cult with a ritual accessory: the yellow band, a.k.a., the Livestrong bracelet. The cancer authorities (in my case, my chemotherapy nurse) dole out these bracelets to patients and loved ones.

I have a Livestrong bracelet. If I am awake and breathing, that son of a bitch is on me—during showers, work, in the gym. I am the man with the yellow band. Live Strong? Hell, yes! I am focused upon survival, and also upon making disparaging comments about cancer. The working title of this book was, in fact, *F_ _ _ Cancer!*

Aside from cancer-club identification purposes, the Livestrong bracelet comes in handy, too, because one of the side effects of my own cancer treatment has been short-term memory loss. I am as flighty as Barbie. I am somewhat surprised that I can even write this book, except that I took copious notes during my treatment. And, for whatever reason, the long-term memory isn't so bad. Just don't ask me why I walked into the room. However, the yellow rubber band hanging off my left wrist reminds me. Here is what it says: You have cancer! Don't give up! Fight! F_ _ _ cancer!"

I happened to read Lance Armstrong's book, *It's Not About the Bike,* before I was ill. When he wrote his memoir, Lance had already attained hero status by winning more Tour de France races than any other man. Now Lance is elevated to superhero because I re-read his book through the eyes of a cancer patient. I want to be like Lance, only without the bike. I don't just want to be *like* Lance, I want to *be* Lance. I want to pummel this nasty invader with exercise and willpower, tenacity and grit and fire. Then I want to move *beyond* Lance and stomp the hell out of cancer, fling its slimy frozen-blueberry nodules from my system, burn them in a fire and destroy the ashes with strong acid so that even my enemies cannot be infected (even if I don't really have enemies). F_ _ _ cancer!

Odds Are You're Fine

I tell Jenelle about my lump and she says nothing at first. But I can read it all in her face: I will die soon and then I will be gone, just like Jim. I can tell what she's thinking: If she says little and is strong, perhaps this will all prove to be a false alarm. If she talks about it too much it might become true, so she says only that it's probably nothing. But her eyes tell me that she does not believe this at all. I don't say much else about it, either. We mention nothing of the lump to the girls and Josefina. We tell ourselves that our lives are so lovely this cannot happen.

I arrive for my Lumpy exam amongst the head colds, odd rashes, and hemorrhoids. Because it is probably nothing, I just drive to my appointment on my own. It is during the work day and work goes on; Jenelle is not available anyhow.

I wait and try to read a *Time* magazine eleven months past its prime, then finally get called to the exam room. I am weighed. I set the scale myself because my weight seldom varies—this precipitates a bit of a turf war when the nurse tries to wrest the counterweight from my hand. "It's okay," I say, "I'm a mechanical engineer." One hundred fifty-five pounds. *Money*. She checks my blood pressure and resting pulse. *Stellar*. This damn lump must be nothing.

I wait some more, then the Physician's Assistant, PA Lucy, comes in. PA Lucy examines Lumpy and feels my throat and asks many questions. She thinks a moment. "Lymph nodes swell for a wide variety of reasons," she says. "It is quite common, in fact."

"Is cancer one such reason?" I say.

"Well, yes," she says, "but there can also be various illnesses, infections, allergies, insect bites—numerous causes."

"Such as cancer?"

"Yes, but we don't know enough to make that call, and judging from your health, age, and the shape you're in, I'd say the odds are quite low that this is cancer."

"Really?" I say, perking up. "Well, I like the sound of that!"

"Yes," she says, "odds are you're fine." But just to be thorough, she orders a full blood workup and an ultrasound of the area to see if this scary entity is, in fact, a swollen lymph node, and perhaps look for any others—possible siblings of Lumpy.

Odds are I'm fine; I feel much better already. I phone Jenelle: "Odds are I'm fine!" We feel much better.

"See?" she says.

I walk straightaway to the ultrasound facility, next to the doctor's office in the same suburban strip center. Long story short: Freezing cold in there, dark in the ultrasound room, slimy goo on the armpit. "Yep," says the technician, "that's a lymph node, all right. But you're not allowed to take my word for it, you have to wait for the official report. Want to see it on the screen?"

This question I find disconcerting. But I stare at Lumpy on the screen. My little baby. Look, you can already make out his face and genitalia! I cannot see the little heart beating, for he has no heart.

I go home and wait. I wait for blood-test results and the official ultra-sound report about Lumpy and Lumpy's possible siblings. I tell Jenelle about the extra testing and offhandedly say, "You know, if the odds are really in my favor, then why are they doing all this extra work?" I am to report back to PA Lucy a week from my initial consultation.

A few days pass and my mental state wavers between calm and panicky. What if it *is* cancer? What if it's *not*? Odds are that I'm fine. What if it is, though? I worry the most at night, in the wee hours of the morning. What if I die at a young age – like my current age? Jenelle says nothing and I feel that it is better this way.

Another day passes and I find what appears to be poison ivy on my back. I do not remember rubbing my back against poison ivy. The rash is mainly on one side. I call the doctor's office and speak with a nurse; she asks if the rash is only on one side. I'm a bit surprised by this question, and say yes, it is. She asks if the rash marks are in any sort of pattern. I say there's a similarity to the Nike swoosh. She says she thinks she knows what it is but will not tell me, as that's up to the doctor or PA Lucy. I move my follow-up visit to the next day so that PA Lucy can tell me what my secret swoosh-rash is.

I take off my shirt in front of PA Lucy. She glances at me for a few seconds, then asks me if I've ever had chicken pox. I say yes.

"You have shingles," she says with a smile.

"Why so happy?" I say. "Granny wasn't very happy when she got shingles."

"Because," she says, "shingles can cause swelling in the lymph nodes."

I ponder this for a split second and my relief comes in a big wave, almost a tsunami. "You mean—"

"Yes," she says. "It's only shingles. Nothing to worry about." She prescribes some exceedingly expensive, non-generic anti-viral shingles medication and sends me on my way. I am ebullient, ecstatic, relieved beyond words to have dodged the Reaper, and also happy that Lumpy will soon subside and leave me for another.

I call Jenelle and we rejoice—I do not have to destroy her by dying so soon after Jim. I call friends and relatives to tell them of my cancer scare and the real cause, which is shingles, and let them know how healthy and happy I am. I take my medication, the shingles disappear, and life is lovely once again.

Months Pass

Months pass serenely. I live a life more peaceful than ever for having dodged death by cancer. I swim, drink coffee, invent interesting equipment for handsome sums of money, and ponder higher levels of existence in the tropical setting of our backyard. Time goes by. Halloween and Thanksgiving come and go, and I have not a care in the world.

Come December, I'm sitting at my desk working away (okay, surfing the web), and notice a bit of numbness down the length of my left triceps. My little voice, which may have been whispering to me for quite some time while I had my fingers in my ears, manages to catch my attention. The voice says, *"Check..."* A moment passes. *"...Lumpy."* Wee Tarzan has startled me by suddenly stepping out from the foliage where he's been exiled. I reach up to my armpit, checking to see if Lumpy has become a flaccid little blueberry raisin on his way back to full domestication. He has not; in fact, he has grown from a blueberry to a frozen grape. *Oh, shit.*

One may read this and say, "Whoa there, buddy! Do you expect me to believe that you were *that* worried and didn't check Lumpy for five months?"

My answer: "Hell yes!" Denial is a powerful force. I did not *want* to check. I wanted to believe.

Anyhow, I call post-haste for a visit, and not with PA Lucy. I call the man himself, the leader of the practice, Doc Savage. Doc Savage does not mince words or miss diagnoses. I hope. I have an appointment for the next day. After the first round, which had nearly devastated Jenelle, I decide to downplay this one. "That damn lymph node still hasn't gone down. I think I'll get it checked just in case." I hope that she will not worry too much. But the look in her eyes tells me that she will.

I arrive and wait for Doc Savage. My weight is taken, sans turf war (155), and my blood pressure checked. No change. I remain the picture of health and athletic virility. Indeed, I would feel quite good about my physique if it were not for Lumpy, the frozen grape.

Doc Savage blows into the examination room, his white coat

ruffling in his wake. "What seems to be the problem?"

I explain my story. He looks like a man who wishes that my story were more concise, yet he listens without interruption. Upon hearing that Lumpy is thriving, he has me remove my shirt and feels under my armpit.

Without the slightest hesitation Doc Savage says, "You need to get that cut out and tested. That could be cancer."

"Whoa, nice bedside manner!" I say. He ignores this and blows out of the room to schedule an immediate appointment with a surgeon. I am left alone with my rapidly accelerating thoughts.

Oh, shit. Lumpy could be cancer, therefore, Lumpy IS cancer! This, I decide, is information I could have used several months prior. Will the delay kill me? Am I a dead man? No, wait, maybe it's not cancer. But maybe....

I tell Jenelle and we repeat the previous dance of strength and silence, but her face, her eyes tell me she is appropriately worried. I pretend not to be. I mean, odds are I'm fine....

Meeting the Surgeon Dude

Doc Savage recommends a surgeon, Doc Young, and so I trust that Doc Young is a good surgeon. Doc Young's practice is in a brand new hospital near my house. It is apparent that this hospital is much-needed; it's just opened and the parking lot is full, already crowded beyond capacity. Doc Young's office is on the fifth floor, affording him a nice view of suburbia. I am given a pre-screening by a nurse with a laptop. What few forms I fill out are scanned and put immediately into the system. Doc Young has computer consoles in each exam room, and also in the room where I am pre-screened by the nurse. He runs a modern, high-tech practice. This I find comforting.

I am led to an examination room and Doc Young arrives. He is younger than me by perhaps ten years. He speaks casually, as if we're going to a kegger, but with medical jargon thrown in. This manner I find less comforting, but he is patient with my questions, willing to explain anything that I want explained, and generally appears quite knowledgeable, dude.

Doc Young explains my procedure and schedules it for his first available opening, a few days hence, on Thursday, December 13. The plan is to have Lumpy removed and sent to the pathology lab for tests. I will not know anything for certain until the results come back from the lab, however long that takes. The biopsy is outpatient surgery; I will be put under for the procedure. Doc Young sends me on my way.

The Biopsy

On the morning of my surgery I am not allowed to eat, which is not a comfortable feeling for me, but it gets worse, as I'm not allowed to drink coffee, either. The thought of people dying while under general anesthesia worms its way into my caffeine-deprived brain and becomes more oppressive than I would prefer. I would prefer this anxiety to be a passing annoyance; instead it threatens to rule my mind. I journal about this before leaving for the hospital: "*. . . in case I don't wake up via some procedural error in my anesthesia . . ..*"

Drama queen? Perhaps. But I can't control the voices in my head. I'm just a reporter.

Jenelle drives me to the hospital; we say nothing. We arrive and check in, and I don the gown. My blood pressure is checked. *Stellar*. This gives me comfort; I could become the healthiest man my anesthesiologist has ever killed. The last few moments before unconsciousness, I feel the drugs working and it feels pretty good—damn good. No worries, dude!

I awaken and we leave, no questions and no discussions, mostly because of the drugs. I remain high all day. The post-surgical pharmaceuticals leave me with a profound serenity, a supreme confidence that the biopsy itself will be the end of all the fuss. Also: I'm pretty sure I can fly.

I nap and by the time I'm awake for dinner, the girls have already eaten. I sit with Jenelle at the dining room table and chow down with my right hand only, which I find amusing. I feel serene and make clever jokes. Vicodin for me is like gin: big drunk; little buzz. It's not too shabby.

Jenelle seems less happy than me, but then again, she is not pharmaceutically prepped for a Grateful Dead concert. Well into the meal, she says "The surgeon..." then stops talking and looks down. Moments pass.

"Surgeon?" I say.

"The surgeon," she repeats, as if that's all I need to know.

"Oh, Doc Young," I chuckle. "Ha, ha, have you heard him talk? Did he call you 'dudette'? Ha, ha."

"Doctor Young," she says without levity, "he talked to me after the operation." She looks down again and takes a breath.

"What is it? We still owe him money? Ha, ha." I serve myself another helping.

She squeezes my hand and looks into my eyes. "He said he couldn't... couldn't get it all out."

"What do you mean? Couldn't get all what out?" I ponder this a moment, but do not understand.

"He says it doesn't look good," she says and starts to cry.

"What? Wait... *what*?" I finally figure out what she's driving at. We end up in each other's arms. I cry, too. My high crashes and everything turns black. It is the end.

2 THE DIAGNOSIS

I am not allowed to raise my left arm higher than my shoulder. I can't sleep on that side. I learn to shower without raising one arm. The bandage is the size of a paperback novel and covers a smaller bandage underneath. There is a lot of swelling within several inches in any direction from the incision. In a couple of days, I am allowed to remove the big bandage, but the smaller one stays. I am not allowed to remove it under any circumstances, and it begins to smell—and not of roses.

I eventually remove the stinky bandage. My armpit is hairless from the operation and a lot of swelling remains. I look at it with a handheld mirror, as I cannot raise my arm high enough to see it in the big mirror. I see the scar, which forms what appears to be a pair of vagina lips sewn together horizontally—a protrusion beneath my arm. The scar disgusts me; the entire region disgusts me. I feel the scar and it remains numb; I cannot feel anything from the scar side of the transaction. I apply Polysporin, rapidly progressing from disgust to nausea. The surgeon has assured me that the skin flap will flatten out with time and look normal, which is good, as I am not fond of having a vagina in my armpit.

Jenelle and I maintain a good front by not talking about my situation to each other or to the girls. Carina and Kaily are happy to assume that I have one of those "Daddy things," like a pulled hamstring or other old-guy ailments or injuries that require no further thought on their part.

Results

It is December 17, and actual results are due today. Even though Doc Young said things didn't look good, I discount his remarks as non-scientific and hold out hope that the pathology proves him wrong. I do not truly believe that he is mistaken, but occasionally find comfort in long-shot optimism. I am, after all, a Cowboys fan.

The sunrise looks like a Salvador Dali painting minus the melting pocket watch and father figure. I take pictures of it. My fate is already determined, and the only thing to do now is become informed. It is out of my hands (I keep telling myself this). The morning is cold and clear; there is frost upon the rooftops. What will be the answer? Maybe nothing until tomorrow, maybe more examinations. Maybe the answer is dire, grim news that will further test my soul. I blame Lumpy for putting me through all of this, the little bastard.

I phone Doc Young's office just after 9:00. Nurse Y answers. She seems reluctant to give me information. I press on. "Look," she says, "if there was bad news the pathology lab would have called immediately."

I pause and try to twist this into good news, but can't get any further than no news. I tell her that the surgeon had discussed additional mass in the region of the lymph nodes. She pauses then puts me on hold so she can speak with him. She comes back on the line and says she'll call the lab to find out about the report. We hang up. I wait.

Nurse Y phones me back. "The lab," she says, "claimed that there is no report and no sample."

"What the hell?"

"Wait," she says, "I'm not finished yet. Doctor Young got on the phone to the lab and said that there darn well is a sample, because he walked it over himself. The lab tech then was able to find the report, and is supposed to fax it over here ASAP."

"What does the report say?"

"We don't know; he'll have to get the fax and read it. Doctor Young will call you back."

We hang up. I wait.

So the lab lost the sample and the report, and I still have no results. I am not filled with confidence in the system. I picture the lab tech making up a report to cover the fact that mine was lost. A dampened anxiety pervades my being. I suddenly feel like the gladiator in the center of the arena, watching the emperor with his thumb out sideways, ready to turn it up or down at whim. I hope that the emperor got some last night. Part of me realizes that the results already exist and that worrying about them will not change a thing. The other part of me wants to scream, cry, punch something, and drive at 150 miles an hour toward El Paso.

My fallback strategy is to exercise. This tactic has served me well for many years as a stress reliever. I arrive at the gym before it occurs to me that I cannot do any upper-body work due to my surgery. Lumpy, you bastard!

I head for the escalator stair machine – in my opinion, the most mentally painful and sweat-producing of all cardiovascular machines. There are various approaches to this machine. A lot of people lean forward and hang off the bars like torture victims who have faith that the batteries must eventually run low in the cattle prod. But I've found that I like to go "no hands" while reading a novel in a proper upright posture. This can be tricky, but allows for a good read.

Today I read *In Cold Blood,* which has been in my gym bag for months. This book is filled with death, and has a familiar character. Lumpy is a psychopath, a drifter; he wants me dead just for the hell of it.

When I am in top form, I can maintain Level 12 or 13 on this stair machine. But it's a mother and induces copious perspiration and hard breathing. This is my first post-surgery workout, so I am glad to set the machine on 9. I go twenty minutes; afterward I stretch my legs and feel a little better about the world and my tenure in it.

I arrive home and shower, still unable to touch the numb lips of the scar without revulsion.

Late in the day, Doc Young has still not returned my call. I phone him and I'm put on hold. The receptionist, not Nurse Y, comes on the line. "Sorry," she says, "but we're closed now."

I have a flash of anxiety that rapidly flares into an abject, unreserved panic. "No! He's supposed to call me!"

"Calm down, sir. Let me take your name." I tell her my name and she pauses. "Oh, sorry, Mr. Baskett. Hold on."

That's more like it.

"Hey," Doc Young says.

"Hey."

"Oh, yeah, well," he says, "sorry it took so long to get back to you."

"That's okay," I say, "I suppose you're pretty busy."

"Oh yeah, I sure am. Buried, you know. You wouldn't believe."

"Hey, I hear you. But anyway, are there any biopsy results yet?"

"Yeah, yeah, the dude just faxed them in." Pause. "The pathology," he says, "is positive."

I let the news soak in with relaxed, closed eyes. "Right on, doc! That's great news!"

"Uhm, well, actually, *negative* would be good."

"But you just said I'm positive!"

"I'm sorry to have to tell you this over the phone, but positive means cancer. The biopsy shows squamous cell carcinoma, metastatic. I've talked to an oncologist and we can get you an appointment right away."

"Whoa, whoa, whoa, what did you just tell me? I have cancer? An oncologist? What did you just say?"

"Squamous cells are the cell type, and metastatic means that the cancer did not originate in your lymph nodes."

I begin to write all this down. "What do you mean it didn't originate there?"

"That means that the cancer has originated elsewhere and has metastasized into your lymph nodes."

"What? Where *did* it originate?"

"I don't know."

"Where else do I have it?"

"I don't know."

"Well, what *do* you know?"

Telling My Family

So now it's official: I have cancer. It's not like I didn't suspect it or have plenty of warning, but I enjoyed brief moments of clinging to small, broken rafts of Styrofoam optimism in a tortured sea of despair. Now the rafts have sunk, which shouldn't happen with Styrofoam. *I have cancer.* The proof: I have an oncologist appointment. I look into the mirror in our master bathroom. I see baldness and withering, pale-skinned death. I am, as they say in Spanglish, *escrewdido*.

I have cancer. See, now I can just blurt that out. Over the years, I've had a tendency to keep my troubles to myself. In a work environment, people would say, "How's it going?"   and I'd say, "Fine" regardless of my actual state (itchy ass, hangover, financial woes, marital strife). "Fine. I'm fine, how are you?"

The word *fine* is fair and reasonable; it doesn't mean *exceptional*. But when I ask how it's going and people answer, "Great!" I know that they are full of shit.

Standard greetings aside, I decide that cancer is not the sort of thing that can be kept as a secret from the family, and *fine* can't reasonably be stretched to cover it. I am suddenly tired of the "I am less affected by the woes of life than you" contest. So I am ready to tell the truth. This new openness policy kicks in moments after getting off the phone with Doc Young.

Jenelle is still at work, so I cannot tell her in person just yet. I call her on the phone. She already knew in that way that wives know things; besides, Doc Young had given a whopper of a hint just after sewing me up. Jenelle cries anyway. I feel badly about telling her the official news, as if I have performed an unconscionable act by getting cancer. We hang up. I go find Kaily to tell her. She is fourteen.

In the late '90s, Carina (ten years old at the time) had a hamster named Cookie. Cookie seemed to be a decent enough hamster except that at a relatively young age, perhaps six months into his new digs at our house, he began to get a brain tumor—on the *outside*. So Cookie would play and frolic and eat and poop and chew things to bits, generally living the dream life of the suburban hamster, but the tumor grew and grew, and eventually became as large as an acorn, then kept growing some more, and came into direct competition with Cookie's original head for size.

I figured that death was imminent, but Cookie lived what I considered an inordinate number of months (or hamster years) with that head-sized tumor hanging out there like Quasimodo's hump, until finally the day arrived when Grimmy came to collect. Cookie dropped dead. He'd been dying for such a long time that Carina seemed to be taking the whole drawn-out demise fairly well. Kaily (five years old at the time) took it equally well.

What is the best and logical thing to do with a dead two-headed pet rodent? "Disappear him" when nobody is watching? Chuck him over the back fence? In retrospect, I endorse that plan wholeheartedly. Instead, I decided to throw a formal hamster funeral. I found a little box; the girls put some cloth in there and laid Cookie's bi-cranial carcass gingerly upon the cloth. This was all jovial enough (the behind-the-scenes jocularity of the funeral parlor) until the actual ceremony.

I picked a burial spot off the back porch and dug Cookie's grave with one of those miniature spades used for flower-pot gardening. Once dirt began to fly, the girls looked at each other and the joviality dried up. Then I laid the box in the hole and improvised a eulogy:

"Cookie was a good hamster; a fine hamster (*despite his disgusting foul tumor the size of a golf ball*), and I for one believe that Cookie is right now on his way to hamster heaven."

Then the tears began. I took a spade full of dirt and was about to toss it onto the box, then paused. Emotions were tenuous, but still somewhat under control.

Well, what is a hamster funeral without a proper closing line? "Earth to earth, ashes to ashes, and dust to dust." I tossed the dirt.

Both girls screamed, then sprinted into the house, slamming the door. The wailing went on for hours, tears flowing, little bodies shaking, and a general cloud of inconsolability. "Cookie! Oh, Cookie!" Snort. "Oh, why?" and that sort of thing. It was as if our whole family, girls aside, had been wiped out by cholera. Then the realization crept in that perhaps I hadn't handled this in the most subtle manner, suitable for small children.

Anyway, you'd think I might have learned something. When I reach Kaily's bedroom, I find her on her bed reading a book, with not a care in the world.

"Hi, Daddy."

"Hi. Hey, listen, I just got off the phone with my surgeon and he had biopsy results."

She looks up at me with an expression that says you're fine, right?

"I have cancer."

This is possibly the number-one crappiest way to break such news to one's young daughter. For the record, I did not pick this method on purpose or with ill intent; I was simply a clueless cancer newbie, not yet the wily veteran cancer-fighting machine who now sits before this keyboard. I had not taken into account that Kaily's life experiences with cancer up until that point had both ended badly: Cookie and Papa Jim. *Daddy makes three.*

I do not know what I am expecting from Kaily at this point, maybe something like, "Oh gosh, sorry to hear that. But do not worry, good father, for together we shall prevail!" Then a supportive hug.

Instead she loses it. "What? No! No! Oh, my God! No! No!" She bolts from the room, runs down the hall, then back up and down the hall, grasping her head and shaking her arms. "No! Oh my God!" She cries, screams, shakes, shrieks toward the ceiling. She is inconsolable.

This is all my fault. Not only will I die soon, I have destroyed my daughter. I am a piece of shit. I should not have gotten cancer, and I should not have told her like this. What have I done?

Jenelle arrives home. Kaily and I are on the couch in each other's arms, Kaily in tears, me pretending to be strong. One moment later, Kaily and Jenelle and I are on the couch in each other's arms, Kaily and Jenelle in tears, me still pretending. But not for long—I cry, too.

Carina is away at Rice University, enjoying her youth without any intimations of mortality. But I have to tell her. I phone her, having rapidly learned some tact from the Kaily incident. I break it to her more skillfully, but it still has to come out. I hear the tears over the phone. Now I have destroyed everyone I love the most. What have I become?

The Next Day

I cannot bear to touch that little sewn-up vagina. I look at it in the mirror, half expecting it to give birth to a seven-pound, twelve-ounce squamous cell.

I have an appointment at 2:00 PM on Tuesday with Dr. Goodcancer, my newly assigned oncologist. I receive a phone call on Monday afternoon.

"Hello, this is Millie at the cancer center."

It's alarming to have people from a cancer center calling for me. Millie informs me that my doctor, whom I haven't seen yet, has been changed. My oncologist is no longer Dr. Goodcancer, but is now Dr. X, and my appointment time is now 11:00 AM. I try to interpret this as some sort of sign, but get nowhere.

* * *

The waiting room at the cancer center is forty by twenty feet, filled with armchairs and couches covered in paisleys and old people. Hanging from one wall is a large LCD television blaring cable news. Nobody is watching. I sit at the end of the waiting room farthest from the TV, but unfortunately I can still hear it. In front of me is a china cabinet seven and a half feet tall, two-thirds empty. It is an odd piece for a cancer waiting room. Disparate curios (a ceramic swan, a crystal vase, a pewter tray, a hospital service award) are arranged on the lower shelves, leaving plenty of space for future randomness higher up. Two of the waiting-room walls are beige; one is yellowish beige, and one is harvest gold. I am without Jenelle because life and work must go on. How do I feel about this? Well, I am being strong; my secret fears and resentments are not allowed to rear their ugly heads. Maybe that means that they do not exist. I've told her I will take notes.

I am the youngest person in the waiting room by perhaps two decades, which explains the volume of the television. The old people complain about traffic, talk amongst themselves, or sit and stare out into eternity. One of the gazers looks at me, perhaps wondering if I am here to pick up my grandfather after his chemotherapy. I nod in acknowledgement of our shared condition. He shakes his head and gazes back out into the void. His look says, "Abandon all hope, ye who enter."

I am called to the desk, and asked for insurance and ID. The identification, I suppose, is so that I don't go beyond the waiting room to where the doctors and poisons are, pretending to be a cancer patient. ("Security! We've got another imposter in here!" Security arrives. "No! No more chemo for you! Quit coming in here!")

In the exam room, a nurse takes my blood pressure. Still stellar. She notes my resting pulse. Sixty. I am, as always, the picture of health and virility. I have no business being in here, except for that scar, the rest of Lumpy, and some of Lumpy's buddies who still reside in my left armpit and are skulking about in parts unknown, ready to annihilate me.

I am left alone for ten minutes to ponder my fate. A woman in a white coat enters the examination room. At first I think that she is yet another nurse who, for some reason, likes to dress as a doctor. This is an attractive woman, perhaps fifteen years younger than I, and that math does not support my idea of a practicing oncologist. But she introduces herself as Dr. X anyway.

I can only stare in shock. I want a seasoned veteran, a wily old "House" sort of character who has seen it all and been there, done that and cured it by ingenious methods. I want experience and field history, and that requires some gray. But I get the attractive young woman.

Dr. X looks over my file. She quickly explains what I've already heard from my surgeon: I have squamous cell carcinoma, metastatic.

"I already know these words, but what I want to know is this: How long do I have to live?"

"Relax," Dr. X says. She explains that squamous cells are native to the throat, lungs, colon, and perhaps a few other places that I forget while trying to ask all the right questions, hear responses, and write everything down, all while pondering the dangers of youth and inexperience. Oh yes, rectum. Squamous cells are found in the pooper.

"So where all do *I* have cancer?"

"Nobody knows."

"Then how can everybody find out?"

Dr. X explains that the full pathology report has not yet arrived, only the preliminary report. The pathology slides will be re-examined by someone higher up the food chain and in a more thorough manner. She prescribes "a full blood workup," a CT scan, and a PET scan.

"What is a PET scan?"

"Positron Emission Tomography," she declaims. This sounds quite scientific and therefore comforting, with an acronym that is somewhat friendly (puppies; very small ducks).

Dr. X explains that a PET scan is similar to a CT scan, except that a nurse will inject me with a vial of radioactive glucose solution one hour beforehand. As it turns out, cancer cells are voracious consumers of glucose, radioactive or otherwise, and so the solution will migrate to the cancer and "light up" on the PET scan results. This scan will tell us how much cancer I actually have. Well, almost. It will tell us how much *detectable* cancer I have, say, any cancerous regions larger than a centimeter (a smallish blueberry, little brother of Lumpy) or perhaps a bit smaller, but not the really tiny ones (fetal Lumpy or his cousin, Sandgrain McLumpy).

I tell Dr. X the story of Jim—how he died of small-cell lung cancer.

"Funny you should mention small-cell lung cancer," she says. "That can look like squamous cells on the slides."

Yeah, I think, *that's a frigging laugh riot.* "So," I say, "lung cancer is on the table as well?"

"Probably not, but it's too early to tell."

Her use of the word "probably" does not comfort me. The word "table" makes me think of our dining room table with one less place setting. Or: a stainless-steel exam table in the morgue.

I ask perhaps fifty questions and take as many notes as I am able to jot down. When there is a lull in our exchange, I look at Dr.

X again. I'm not known for my tact to begin with, but in matters of life and death, especially my own, I can be virtually tact-free.

"Look," I say. "You seem to be quite knowledgeable, and excuse me for saying this, but your age... I have to tell you, it scares the hell out of me. Could you... can you give me some comforting words about your background? You look like the ink on your diploma is still wet."

As the words finish leaving my mouth, my brain kicks in, late as ever, and says, *Are you insane? This doctor may be your only hope! Don't piss her off before she even does anything!* One of my (perhaps many) other voices says, *Screw that! Get an older one and live longer! Bail out, now!* Dr. X gives me a curious look, but nowhere in her demeanor do I sense anger or even crumbs of annoyance. "It's okay," she says, "I get that all the time." She goes on to tell me about her medical school, her internship, her years of experience, and how Dr. The Man (whom I haven't met yet, but who built and runs this particular cancer center) hand-picks his staff. Her pedigree is, indeed, top-notch, tempered by big-city, brand-name cancer hospital experience.

I calm down. "Sorry," I say, "it's just that I expected... well, a little gray."

She smiles. "Don't worry," she says, "you're in good hands."

I experience a brief moment of serenity. I believe her. Maybe. But there is no time for further misgivings, as there are tests to be run and blood samples to be drawn.

I am told to walk directly across the lobby to schedule PET and CT scans as soon as there are openings. This is refreshing–from a "let's get this show on the road" perspective–and terrifying, from a "you don't have a moment to lose" perspective. I receive one form for the scans and two forms for blood, which is to be sucked from a vein immediately after I schedule my scans.

In the scan office, an elderly Hispanic woman listens to my plea for scheduling and looks over my paperwork. It seems to confuse her, but she takes my identification and insurance, typing the information into her computer nonetheless. She carries my paperwork into the back and returns thirty seconds later, types some more at her computer. She takes my paperwork into the back one more time, returning five minutes later.

"No can I schedule appointments in here." She points out a number on the form and says, "This number you must call."

"But you do the scans in here?"

"Yes," she says, "we do scans here."

"But you can't schedule the scans?"

"No," she says. "This number you must call."

"But Dr. X said to walk over here and schedule this myself."

"Let me see this paper," she says. "I will ask in the back."

"No, no, no, I'll just call."

I walk outside the scan office and call the number using my cell phone. After several rings a scheduling desk somewhere in the bowels of the cancer center or Mumbai answers. They schedule my scan for tomorrow, December 19.

There are three elevators in the medical center lobby, and a line of people waiting to ascend. A car arrives and the bell dings; people begin to file in. In my current mood I'm not fond of crowds, so I run up the stairwell to the second floor where the blood lab awaits its victims. As I pass the elevator it dings and opens. I walk extra fast, and quite a few people file out from the elevator car. But I am one step ahead, which gives me a momentary satisfaction. I submit my paperwork and I'm rewarded with more paperwork. I am asked for my identification ("No, imposter! No more blood drawings for you!") and insurance again, and told to take a seat.

The waiting room is full of people of all ages. The building is not just a cancer hospital; it houses all sorts of doctors, many of whom like to draw blood from their patients. The TV blares cable news; perhaps two people watch.

At last my name is called and I'm led to the blood-letting seat, a padded vinyl affair, extra wide for the new stout Americans, and with foldable arms on either side for righties and lefties. I am a righty. The phlebotomist (I love that word) robotically asks me how I am.

"So far, so good. Well, other than the cancer thing."

She doesn't seem to hear, and instead dabs some gauze in alcohol, ready to swab my arm.

She stops, frozen, startled. "Oh, my!" she says.

"What? What is it?" A tumor? Lumpy on the move?

"Your veins!" she says.

A leak? "What is it?" I look down at my veins and back up.

She makes full eye contact. "Oh, those are nice... mmm, mmm, mmm..."

I am a pork chop and she's a starving lion. "I have nice... veins?"

"Oh, yes, honey. Those are fabulous!"

I perk up. I feel pride. Nobody has ever complimented my veins before. Blood will be drawn, but through an admired vein.

"So, I take it from your comment that nice veins aren't always the case?"

"Hardly ever see 'em," she says. "Sometimes I can't even find 'em!"

She applies the tourniquet and her eyes grow another notch. I think I see saliva forming and teeth beginning to point. The needle hits the vein on the first touch. Dark crimson fills two vials.

Phone Calls

Time passes. Notifications are passed along to friends and family. My house and cell phones ring at all hours; my email beeps. People want updates; they want to talk at length, and often. I am touched; I had no idea that people cared so much, and it makes me feel warm inside. I have no privacy. The phone rings, and rings some more.

I ponder composing a cheery holiday update via e-mail: *Yes, it's Christmas again, and the family is doing great. I have a little cancer and don't know how long I have left, but we are so blessed to find out that I have nice veins.* Instead, I keep it sincere and gentle, and thank everyone for their concern. I politely request that the Concerned limit their phone calls because I cannot take many more of them, lest I spontaneously combust.

Even so I continue to tell more people about my cancer. I call Master Steel Curtain, my taekwondo instructor, who is also a good friend.

Master SC is shocked. "You're too healthy to have cancer!"

"Yeah, how do you think I feel about it?"

He insists on helping. I explain to him that I'm only telling certain individuals at this point, especially at his school, because I don't want to feel like a cancer-freak/charity case to be stared at or treated with kid gloves—the weakest member of the athletic herd, ready to be culled.

"I don't think that would happen," he replies. But I remain unconvinced and ask him to keep the news to himself.

* * *

It is one month until my forty-fourth birthday. It occurs to me that I will still be alive by then. That I would even consider that it could be otherwise speaks of the dark thoughts going through my head. Unbidden thoughts come in the night, usually around four AM—thoughts of death and fear and *"if I had only..."* (*made a will, been nicer, not studied engineering, dated so-and-so in 1981*). Was Lumpy caused by the car painting I did in high school and college? Those lacquers and solvents and fumes that made my muscle cars shiny? From drinking too much? Is it liver cancer? Pancreatic cancer? Am I dead in ninety days? I do not know how much cancer I have, only that it is metastatic and of the squamous variety. Whenever I Google the topic it scares the hell out of me, so I try to avoid Googling, period.

3 TESTING, TESTING

Cancer has lousy timing. Jenelle and I happened to spend all our liquid cash to move into a junior McMansion just one month and ten days prior to my diagnosis. Our new house sits on a golf course; we gave up our pool and affordable monthly note to get it. Our previous house was one-third paid for and certainly would have taken care of our needs into old age. We could have afforded the note on Jenelle's salary alone, if for some odd reason I could no longer work. Now we have a more expensive house and no savings to speak of, and I have cancer. As it turns out, having cancer is not inexpensive.

So I wonder: Will Jenelle abandon the new place if I keel over? I have a decent amount of life insurance, so she could pay it off. She likes the house, but I've seen women flee once the husband dies. After my father-in-law died, my mother-in-law moved. After my maternal grandfather died, my grandmother left the farm so fast I think the skid marks are still at the end of the driveway. Will Jenelle move? Will I die? Yes, but I don't know when.

Other fun cancer timing involves health insurance. In a normal year, we never come close to spending our insurance deductibles. But cancer burns through deductibles like bottle rockets through gym shorts. So we enjoy the double bonus of spending the '07 deductibles between mid-December and New Year's, then spending the '08 deductibles before the ink is dry on the new calendar. It turns out that our health-insurance deductibles are a few thousand dollars per family member per year. Holy double-dipping deductibles, Batman! Cha-ching!

* * *

I take a shower, during which I feel that I will undoubtedly die soon and so all of that money business will soon be OPP (Other People's Problems). During that thought, I experience the luxurious warmth of the water. I realize, after nearly forty-four years, that a simple hot shower is one of life's exquisite pleasures. I decide on the spot that I want to soak up as many of life's exquisite pleasures as I can in the time that I have left.

After a few moments of bliss, I look up at the ceiling, perhaps for guidance from above, and spy the extra shower head. This is the first house I've lived in where the master shower has two heads. Head number two is the size of a pie pan and filled with little nozzles, perhaps one hundred of them. It hangs eight feet above the floor and looks like it will provide an additional gentle spray of hot water, which might really hit the spot. I turn the valve for number two.

Water floods out at an absurd number of gallons per second and, as it turns out, at the same temperature as Lake Superior in April. After my screams, the water warms up and I peel myself from the shower wall. I have to say, the decadent fat-cat two-shower-head bourgeoisie are onto something. Oh, the flow!

The PET Scan

I report to the waiting room of the scan department. A PET scan does not seem to demand my wife's presence, and so I am alone again. Sometimes I wish I were not, but I am strong and tough, and life goes on. The same older Hispanic woman tends the department's desk. She smiles and hands me paperwork to fill out: various release-of-liability forms, directives to pull the plug in the event of a long-term coma, and a form to list my medications and medication allergies. This last form is filled with blank lines, perhaps thirty of them.

"Whoa," I say, "look at all these spaces for medications!"

"Is okay," she says. "A second form I can give you if this one you fill up."

I find a small box off to the side that says "no medications" and check that one. I sign the rest of the forms without reading them and hand them all back.

"Thank you, Mr. Hewitt," she says.

I explain that I am not Mr. Hewitt and pre-empt her next request by handing her my driver's license and insurance card.

"But," she says, "your name is not the name which the computer tells me."

"Well, my correct name is the one on my driver's license."

She stares at me as if I am speaking Martian. At last she snaps out of her trance; time passes as she makes three phone calls to straighten the problem out. She finally believes that I am not Mr. Hewitt and begins to enter the information from my insurance card.

Jenelle is the one with health insurance. The old Hispanic woman enters information for several minutes, then asks me if Jenelle is the name of my company.   "No," I say.

She looks confused, but keeps typing. Perhaps three minutes later she stops typing and says, "Then who is this Jenelle?"

A patient (seventy-something white guy) comes in and sits near me, but does not look up and says nothing.

A doctor passes through, pauses, looks at me and says, "Hello, sir!"

"Hello, doctor, sir!"

The TV blares, but nobody watches it. I glance up and see that it is tuned to a soap opera. A woman speaks with her husband; she looks earnestly into the camera. "Thank you," she says, "for being a horndog and a lush." For a second, I think she is speaking to me, but snap out of it when I am called to the back.

The PET-scan people have their own vein specialist, Ms. Pet Scan, an attractive young woman hauling a cart of various needles and solutions. Ms. Pet Scan throws out some garden-variety, make-the-patient-relax banter (*How are you today? Is this your first time?*) before getting down to business. She places my arm on the pad and prepares to swab it.

"Ooh, oh, my!" she says. "You've got those textbook veins!" Her eyes reveal unbridled vein lust. She looks into my eyes and then back at my veins.

"I'm starting to get that a lot," I say.

"I'll bet you do!"

I feel like a porn star at a fan-club meeting. *Tourniquets are applied. Veins throb. Phlebotomists swoon.*

Ms. Pet Scan takes a small dab for a blood-sugar test. It turns out my level is spot-on, right in the middle of the desirable range. I am as healthy as a young Charles Atlas. Except for this cancer thing. She injects me with saline solution from a plastic syringe, then disappears and returns with a small metal lock-box the size of a toaster. The box has a "Danger! Radioactive!" sticker on it with the corresponding symbol. Ms. Pet Scan pulls a stainless syringe from the box and injects me with the radioactive goo. I don't know what radioactivity is supposed to feel like, but I experience some pressure in my vein.

"Will I glow in the dark?"

"I get that a lot," she says.

"I'll bet you do!"

I am escorted to my own private waiting chamber. There is a large radiation sign on the door, which I realize is not about the room—it is about *me*. The room is twelve feet long by five feet wide with a ten-foot ceiling. The floor is linoleum—one-foot squares in various hues last popular in the 1970s. Inside the room a TV blares. Ms. Pet Scan hands me the remote and I turn the TV off.

"Most people leave it on," she says.

I shrug. There is a Lazy-Boy recliner that looks inviting. Ms. Pet Scan asks if I want some water.

"Hell, yes, I want some water!"

I explain that I've had no food or drink since 9:00 PM the night before, per the PET scan scheduler's instructions.

"You mean to tell me she didn't let you drink water?"

"That's exactly what I mean to tell you. If you pull out a bottle of water, I'll look at it like you just looked at my veins."

She walks off and comes back with a cool bottle of water. I down it in one long chugalug. "You don't have any coffee back there, do you?" I ask. She smiles.

Ms. Pet Scan brings me a white cotton blanket and turns off the light. I wonder if she might wish to hang out with me and watch my veins while I sleep, but she closes the door and leaves instead. There is a single window in the wall by the door overlooking the corridor. It is covered by a drawn mini-blind. I hear people talking through the glass.

I ponder a phone conversation I had the night before with a friend. He said: "Don't bring your dog to the PET scan, and don't bring your cat to the CAT scan!" We had a good laugh on that one. He also said that if I begin treatment anywhere else, MD Anderson won't touch me. I drift off to sleep.

It takes one hour for radioactive goo to become lunch for Lumpy and his offspring.

A knock at the door wakes me. Ms. Pet Scan escorts me—groggy, caffeine deprived, and radioactive—to the dimly lit den of the PET scan machine. I am told to remove my shirt and everything from my pockets. The machine is a large white donut, perhaps six feet in diameter and four feet long, with a human-sized hole in the middle. A long, slim platform resembling a narrow bed on a conveyor belt feeds the maw. I look for the placard that says this scanner was built by the Freud corporation.

Ms. Pet Scan has me lie on the bed, face up. While I'm getting comfy she tells me I'll have to drop trou (which I will have to repeat for all scans).

"Uhm, while I'm laying down?"

"Yep!"

Note that I have cancer, I am in a cancer hospital to engage in a life-and-death battle, and I am tended to by medical professionals, so what does Ms. Pet Scan do? She holds up a cotton sheet so that I can drop trou without any embarrassment from someone spotting my tighty whities. Afterward, the scan technician and Ms. Pet Scan position my arms over my head, and prop my knees up on a foam pillow. The sheet covers everything but my face, as I am not dead yet. All personnel leave the room.

There is a moment of calm; then the gurney begins to move and I am slowly fed into the big white tube.

A round wall of white surrounds me. I see...dead people? Heaven? Myself as a five-year-old pulling Granny Baskett's freshly planted flowers one at a time from the loamy bed? No, I see screws—a smattering of stainless, Phillips head screws that hold the plastic cover onto the inside of the scanner. I can see a narrow translucent band, perhaps one-inch wide, which encircles the tube just inside the entrance. Behind the band a few red lights flash. The ring begins to move with the subdued sound of a massive turbine spooling up all around me.

The turbine attains its medical RPM and a Pink Floyd song begins inside my head: *Welcome my son, welcome to the machine....*

Welcome to the cancer machine, the fearful scanner, the life or death machine.

In various time increments—from a few seconds to a few minutes—the bed stays still, scoots further into the tube, a bit out of the tube, and back into the tube so far that my head pokes out the other end while they scan "the naughty bits." I hope they don't find any cancer in *those*. The turbine whirs; thoughts spin. The scan looks into me, through me, God-like, seeing things about me that I cannot see myself—or won't.

How is my marriage really? Am I who I want to think I am?   Will I die or live? Is my cancer everywhere? Coffee... I need coffee....

The scan machine abruptly disgorges me and the technician tells me over the speaker that I can pull my pants up. There hasn't been any physical penetration, so why do I feel a bit like Ned Beatty after the hillbilly finished with him?

After the scan I cannot go home and glow in the dark just yet. I must first walk over to the other side of the cancer facility and pick up "contrast" for tomorrow's CT scan. Contrast is non-radioactive goo that I must drink to make Lumpy show up well against all the armpit bits that aren't trying to kill me (I hope he shows his good side).

A girl behind the counter holds up two jugs of contrast. "You want banana or berry?"

"I'll take berry," I say, "I hear it's berry delicious!"

The girls behind the counter laugh. I am happy to be so entertaining while suffering. While I wait for my contrast goo, I take a seat in the waiting area. The TV blares; no one watches. One black couple, one thirty-something Asian guy, one old white guy, and one Hispanic couple all sit, waiting for something. That's what I love about cancer: no discrimination!

I spot a coffee machine and lunge for my first cup of the day. The coffee is fairly rank by normal standards, but especially rank considering how much money flows through this place. However, it *is* coffee, and I find comfort in that.

CT Scan

I shower, gritting my teeth to wash the scar. During the lovely warm flow of the two-headed shower, I recall that there are not many shopping days left until Christmas. I need to figure out how to shop for Jenelle and the girls in the midst of scans and tests that will confirm whether this is my last holiday shopping season.

I slept better last night, without awakening at four AM to worry about mortality, a notable achievement. Also notable at this moment is diarrhea, induced by drinking one and a half jugs of berry delicious "Readi-Scan 2" (the sequel) dye. I am obliged to save the other half jug to chugalug right before my appointment.

I exercised last night while Kaily was at taekwondo class. I can no longer attend with her because of my Lumpy-ectomy. Instead I went to the gym and did twenty minutes on the escalator stair machine, then leg weights and stretching. I worked up a sweat, and it felt good.

Afterward, I went to the *do-jang* to pick Kaily up, and one of my fellow students, Mrs. C, gave me a hug with a look of empathy that one might give to a man who won't be around for another hug. She didn't say anything, but I assume that Master Steel Curtain had spilled the beans, as this is not her usual behavior.

* * *

When Jenelle and I next talk, we discuss logistics—what scans or tests are coming up, when the appointments are, will I be okay on my own for each one, etc. We don't go into much depth. Depth is scary, like opening the wrong manhole cover, the one that happens to be a portal to hell. You leave that manhole closed.

I do not want to dredge up Jenelle's grief over Jim's death, and I get the feeling that neither does she. I mostly keep all my doubts and fears inside except when I journal. Every once in a while I tell Jenelle I am scared, and she admits that she is, too. Neither one of us says anything to the girls. I honestly don't know how they are affected and try to maintain a strong front, propping up the myth that their father is a superman to whom no harm can come. I like to think that Kaily buys it. When Carina calls to check up on me, we focus on logistics—like mother, like daughter. I go to my CT scan alone.

Cars and trucks on the freeway are backed up, as usual, to *Viejo Carajo*. It has been a while since I've participated in rush-hour traffic due to my mellow, pool-gazing consultant lifestyle, and I feel out of practice. I would prefer to be airlifted by helicopter. I pull into the cancer center for my CT scan at 7:27. Fear breeds punctuality.

First stop: a unisex restroom in the main corridor of the radiology wing. The stainless steel trash can overflows with paper towels, the sink is wet, and the floor has small bits of toilet paper (not used) lying about. It reminds me of a McDonald's restroom I visited once near Waco during a hurricane evacuation.

The radiology waiting-room carpet is dark blue with a nausea-inducing pattern of light blue and copper; the walls are pale yellow. The furniture is covered in two distinct and non-complementary fabrics (contemporary pattern of yellow with orange and blue southwestern colors, and dark green with a grandmotherly floral pattern). Most of the chairs are supersized. The TV blares. One man, a fifty-something white guy, watches the morning news. A fifty-something Hispanic man appears to be in shock, having taken a long look under the wrong manhole cover.

The weather is pleasantly warm for December, hot almost, but I failed to bring a jacket for indoors. All enclosed Texan environments are chilled beyond reason by large-tonnage air conditioning systems anytime the thermometer rises outside. I sit across from the door to the Great Hall of Zaps and wait, hugging myself for warmth.

An African-American fellow the size of an NFL lineman sits beside me. He introduces himself in a deep baritone as Mr. J. "What are you here for?" he asks.

I tell him about my diagnostic CT scan for cancer. He nods and tells me of his own testicular cancer a few years back.

"Hey, that's like Lance Armstrong!"

"I know," he says. Mr. J recounts his treatment and explains that he had to have one testicle removed in 2000. "My wife," he says, "was diagnosed with breast cancer right after I finished treatment. She died two years later." He tells me that he is in remission and that he hears peach pits are good therapy.

"Are you here for a follow-up?" I ask.

"No, I was lifting a door and hurt my back."

"That must have been some heavy door to hurt *your* back."

"Well," he says, "it was made of lead."

"You lifted it by yourself?"

"Yeah."

I nod, and we both stare at the carpet a moment. "Why were you lifting a lead door by yourself?"

"It's for another hospital, for the radiology department."

So here we are, seven years after Mr. J's cancer treatment, and he looks as healthy as can be and is lifting lead doors, with just one peach pit at that! This gives me comfort.

Mr. J is called in for his scan; he shakes my hand and leaves. I amazed to learn so much about a man within moments of meeting him. This turns out to be the way it is with cancer—it's a common bond and we club members come to realize how important it is to share our experiences, to know we are not alone. Also, once you give death serious consideration, it's hard to give a rat's ass about formality.

I get the call. Entering the Great Hall of Zaps, I am guided to a locker room and strip down to a surgical gown. After emerging I'm led to a trolley before the CT scan machine. At first glance, the CT scan machine looks a lot like the PET scan machine. A technician asks me which side I prefer for the IV. Surprise me, I say. He picks the right arm, the same as all the other vein pokers thus far. He plugs the IV in without complimenting my veins and I feel insulted. My IV needle is attached to a tightly coiled hose, akin to a telephone cord. The other end of the telephone cord is attached to an electronic dispenser filled with iodine solution. The technician leaves and enters the control room. The trolley electronically guides me into the tube.

From a speaker inside the tube, the technician asks if I'm ready for the iodine. "You may feel a little heat sensation," he says.

I tell him I'm ready and he pushes a button. A warm flow of iodine caresses my testicles for a brief moment. I experience a combination of fleeting euphoria and a feeling that I've peed all over myself. Then I decide that one doesn't necessarily preclude the other, and enjoy the feeling all the more. But it passes, and I remain dry and no longer euphoric. The warm, piss-like testicle caress becomes the most memorable sensation of my CT scans. Other memorable aspects include the long phone-cord-like umbilical to the iodine injection unit, hums and whirs, stainless-steel screws, and IV tape pulled off with arm hair attached.

A Sign

On the evening of my first CT scan, the weather cools to perfection and I open the house windows for a bit of fresh air. I feel fit and life seems normal. Kaily is okay and Jenelle is okay, and I wander into the master bedroom. The lights are off. The window screens are low, and I find myself on my knees, looking out into the darkness. Behind our house the golf course is two fairways wide, and there are few lights visible from the houses across the way.

The sky is clear and beautiful, a deep indigo. I ponder the scans of the last two days and wonder if I will have the strength to deal with all of this. I find that the individual procedures are not so arduous on their own, but they have a cumulative effect on my psyche, each a brick of worry in a growing wall of foreboding. The waiting, the unknown—these are the real challenges.

Our house lies on the outer fringe of a flight pattern from Houston Intercontinental Airport. At certain hours under certain wind conditions, the odd passenger jet flies overhead. I see landing lights blinking off in the distance. The cool quiet evening envelops me, and I realize that I appreciate it more intensely than usual. I embrace the moment and let it course through me.

The landing lights draw near—so near that they become a distraction. It appears that the plane will fly directly over our house. It's flying so low, so fast! The lights streak over the golf course and, as they whip past, I see a trailing light, the color of green fireworks. The light moves far too quickly for an airplane and I realize that there is no noise—no propeller, jet thunder, or any sound whatsoever. I decide that this is some sort of sign—a falling star—and wish upon it. I wish for life.

December 21, 2007

I called Dr. X yesterday. Actually, I did not call her. In order to reach Dr. X, I dialed the phone number for the cancer practice. No other humans were involved in the interchange:

Welcome to the cancer practice. If you are a doctor or an insurance carrier press one, if you are a patient, press two.

I note that insurance companies rank higher than patients.

For Doctor A, press one; for Doctor B, press two; for Doctor C, press three; for Doctor X, press four. If you need to speak to Doctor X, press one; if you would like to leave a message with Doctor X's nurse, press two. Hello, you have reached the voice mailbox of Dr. X's nurse. If you would like to leave a message, please wait until the tone, then leave your name, date of birth, and brief message, including your return telephone number. Someone will attempt to call you back within the same business day. If it is after three PM, you may not be called back until the next business day. Beep!

"Uhm, yes, I'm hemorrhaging blood through all of my God-given orifices and also two new ones. Oh, and my vaginal underarm scar just gave birth to a seven-pound, twelve-ounce squamous cell named LJ, for Lumpy Junior. It's after three, so I guess I'll just sit here by the phone until tomorrow."

Okay, this is what I really said: "Hi, this is David Baskett, one of Dr. X's patients. I'm waiting for PET scan results and CT scan results, and I was hoping to speak to a human about all of this, but that doesn't seem to be one of my menu choices.... So maybe you could call me back? My number is 555-5555. Okay, please call back!"

I wait. Time passes. Jenelle calls from work, urgent to hear the news, but I have none.

I kill time by looking in the mirror. I lift my left arm until it hurts. I've regained about a third of my pre-surgery range of motion. I cannot decide if this is a positive sign, but chalk it up to progress nonetheless. I kill more time by lying on the floor of the office. I kill even more by looking out the window at the golf course—weeds, dead grass. I wait all day.

Finally I wade back into Dr. X's phone menu at 2:50 PM. Beep! I leave my message again. More waiting.

It is after 4:00 PM when I give up hope of hearing news. At last, the phone rings. "Hello?" I say.

"David? This is Dr. X's nurse."

"Oh, hi! How are you?"

"I'm returning your call."

"Yes, I'm hoping to hear my PET scan and CT scan results."

"Well, about that," she pauses. "It is the holiday season, you know. I apologize but the radiologist who normally provides the evaluation, well, it is nearly Christmas and I apologize, but he won't... there won't be any results available until December twenty-seventh."

"What? The twenty-seventh? I have to go through Christmas like this?"

Here is some sage cancer advice: Do not get diagnosed during the holiday season unless you like suspense.

* * *

While I await December twenty-seventh, I experience small aches here and there and decide that they are cancer. I feel my whole body for lumps. I've never done this much global lump exploration before and, as it turns out, there are a few oddly shaped bits scattered about, especially in my abdomen. I stop and take calming breaths. I feel my abdomen again. I feel the region just south of my sternum where the lower-most ribs converge.

There is a low-level discomfort in this region, and a formation that is definitely, possibly lumplike. I haven't looked up where the pancreas is, or even so much as a spleen, but I feel that this must be my pancreas.

This odd bit of flesh has probably been here all along, but at this moment it is the vanguard of an army of Lumpy's cousins, in-laws, and countless illegitimate spawn. They are all humping like rabbits in order to take over my body with a cancerous population boom. I experience a slight ache in a different region near my stomach: must be cancer. There is a slight scratchiness in my throat: probably cancer. This is all giving me a headache. Brain cancer! I am rife with slimy death cells and tumors of all sizes and shapes. I will die before I hear my PET scan results on December 27...

Be a man! I tell myself.

I am a man, a dead man.

Shut up!

You shut up!

Mom!

The argument going on in my head makes me batty, so I decide to go to the gym. Before I go, I walk out back and gaze upon the golf course. I glance down at the yellowed St. Augustine grass and find Bonehead's throw toy, unused for weeks. Why not? I think, and give it a toss across the yard. She sprints, grinning her Golden Lab grin—instant rapture—then fetches the toy and charges back directly toward me. For years we've played our special game: she fetches then sprints past me, knowing I will try to catch her.

She jukes at the last moment but I juke as well, nearly grabbing the throw toy as she runs past. This makes me happy, as stealing anything from Bonehead's mouth entails no small degree of athleticism.

She walks over, victorious, and drops the toy at my feet. I give it another toss, farther this time. She races past, this time on my left side—the Lumpy side—and I reach out, over-extending my arm and, hence, my surgery site. I feel a sharp pain and wonder if I've just ripped my vagina lips open. I withdraw to the house, dejected and sore. But at least I'm not bleeding.

I set the escalator stair machine on level twelve for twenty minutes. At minute eleven, it occurs to me that I am not having a good time. In fact, if I were to do such a thing on a regular basis it would put me off exercise entirely. This is anti-fun. However, I reckon that a stint on an escalator stair machine will be one of the more pleasurable uses of time available to me in the ensuing months, what with all the radiation, chemotherapy, and God knows what else I'll have to endure. There is time for reflection during the escalator machine—hours, it seems, as the minutes grind by—and I try to use this time to inure myself to suffering. So far I have suffered without attaining inurement.

With sweat pouring and lungs burning, I devise a theory: The mechanism for a PET scan is to supply cancer cells with radioactive glucose because cancer cells are voracious consumers of glucose. Ergo, if I use up all my normal glucose via exercise, I'll starve the little bastards! If I have groups of cancer cells crying out for nutrients, but have much larger groups of muscle cells using up the fuel, then the muscles win.

On the other hand, my muscle/glucose theory could be complete crap. I was in good shape *before* being diagnosed; how come the theory didn't work then? But who says it didn't? I might be dead right now if I hadn't been exercising so much *before.*

I take a vote, and my arguing voices concur upon two points: One, the theory has some holes in it. Two, the theory makes me feel better and gives me some hope. And it certainly can't hurt to be in good shape during cancer treatment. The motion carries: I will exercise like a demon while I can.

The stair machine is followed by a solid leg workout (almost back to full strength on the various machines). Maneuvering gingerly onto the bicep machine, I find that I need not put any shoulder into the exercise if I keep the weights light. I do a delicate set. Same with the triceps machine. Things are looking up. The ab work feels good! Oh, excuse me, Lumpy, are you getting hungry? Die, little bastard!

A brief period of calm ensues. I take inventory. My lungs feel like they are working at full capacity. I do have a slight cough—it has just emerged in the last several days. I still have a slight ache in the abdominal cavity. The voice of fear says it's all cancer and the voice of reason calmly explains that the cough is probably due to the epic stress of my situation. I vote with reason.

Carina is home from Rice for Christmas break. She and Kaily seem to enjoy seeing me return from the gym; surely that means all is well. How else could the old man sweat like that? I wonder if Jenelle will buy in, but her eyes say no. We go to bed.

Christmas Eve, 2007

It is 12:40 AM. Presents are wrapped, daughters are sleeping. I drink Johnny Walker Black and check for lumpiness in my abdominal cavity. I probe just beneath where my ribs come together and the terrain feels lumpy and hard. I wander over to the window and stare up at the moon's dispassionate glow. Perhaps the moon knows how all this will end.

"Merry Christmas," I say. The moon doesn't reply.

I allow myself a fifty percent chance that this will not be my last Christmas on this Earth. I generously give myself a ninety-nine percent chance of seeing my forty-fourth birthday, as it's coming next month. I give up one percent because, well, shit happens.

Jenelle and I have a Christmas Eve tradition of drinking Scotch or Irish whiskey, depending on the mood. After the presents are wrapped, we kick back and speak nostalgically of the previous year and how lucky we are, how great the girls are. Jenelle comes in with her drink, looking for a ribbon. The Johnny Walker works its magic and I forget about the real or imagined lumps for a moment and smile at her. I think back to our summer vacation and how well my consulting firm has done.

"You know," I say, "2007 has been a pretty good year."

Jenelle looks over and starts crying.

Oh, shit. "Uhm, other than *that*, I mean." Oops. F-ing cancer! F_ _ _ cancer!

I've pretty much ruined the mood, so I apologize and go upstairs to journal about my feelings. Journaling is my version of "In case of emergency, break glass." Here is what I write:

Pancreatic cancer? I should start a pool. Take bets. Instead of drawing squares, we could draw regions of the anatomy or internal organs. I don't even know what a pancreas does. Pancreates, I suppose. It's all very odd, writing as a potential dead man—I mean, if there's a chance I'll fight like hell, but there may not be a chance. Thursday, Dr. X may tell me to put my affairs in order. And if she does, I'll likely be distressed, yet not overtly surprised.

Christmas Morning

My daughters give me a joint present—a large frame holding nine snapshots. The snapshots were taken on our family vacation in Ireland in the summer of 2007, just before I found Lumpy the first time (oh, they grow up so fast). I look at myself in the photographs—the very picture of naive bliss, vivacious, joyful. I am moved that my girls have created this set of photos, but find these images cruelly ironic. I peek at the photos again. Those were the good old days. So contented, so unknowing, so recent.

The whole family scrambles into the car, and we drive north to visit family. This year's destination is my sister's house in South Lake, an affluent McMansion paradise northeast of Ft. Worth, complete with a brand-new "old town" square. There, we open presents and try to find Christmas joy while we feast on tender roast beef. I do not know if I am imagining things, but I feel like the elephant in the room that people strive not to recognize.

I escape to the backyard and climb onto the trampoline. I bounce over the brown winter lawn in the crisp air, looking out over farmland beyond the back fence. I bounce around to face the house. I can see through the window into the den, where my parents, siblings, offspring, and nieces and nephews have gathered. I jump high to show them how virile and healthy I am. They stare out at me with blank expressions. They are staring at the poor sickly relative who apparently plans to expedite his death via trampoline.

December 26

It's dark already and traffic is thick. Jenelle is at the wheel because we believe that this will be less stressful for me. Instead, it gives me time to feel trapped and out of control. From the passenger seat I cannot control our car, just as I cannot control my life or fate or Lumpy.

By the time we pull into the driveway, I have conducted enough ugly internal dialogues to drive my stress level into the red. For a good portion of the drive I've been quiet, and when I am quiet Jenelle is quiet, perhaps thinking that this will keep me calm. We drag into the house and I hope that I can somehow calm down. It is at this moment that Kaily vociferously complains about the smell.

I left a full trash bag in the kitchen can, and it has come of age. Kaily complains again; it does not occur to her to solve the problem by taking the trash out herself. She has an alternate solution: she digs up a spray can and proceeds to perfume the kitchen air. Unfortunately for all involved, what happens next precipitates what I like to call "a scene."

Kaily accidentally sprays me in the face. I finally lose it. "Don't spray that on me! What the hell are you thinking? Just take the damn trash out!" Kaily cries—it's not just the words I use, but the eyes and intonation, the caustic disapproval and rage—like the bad old days before my consulting firm.

Jenelle gives me "the look" (which in my head translates to "You are pond scum, you low-life psychotic bastard!") and Carina can't stand all the turmoil and runs up to her room and slams the door. Fearing my own emotions, I grab my gym bag and flee. Thank God our local gym is open all hours, because it is 10:30 PM, the day after Christmas.

I work out, putting in my twenty-minute session on the escalator machine. I do an arm workout slightly more rigorous than the previous one, plus thirty crunches and a full set of leg weights, followed by stretching. I sweat a lot. The stress begins to recede ever so slightly.

Back home, I apologize to everyone. Out of pity, I suppose, they accept my litany of "sorries." I blame cancer for the whole incident. In all the noise of the evening, I fail to make the connection between the fact that I will be getting my scan results tomorrow and the way my emotions are puking all over the place.

D-Day: December 27

The sun rises as I peruse the grocery list on the fridge: beer, wine, trash bags, toilet paper. I feel like adding "last will and testament." This thought does not provide a jumpstart for the day. But when I reach up for a coffee mug, the very first one my eyes fall upon says "Live." This is one side of the "Live, Love, Eat" mug, another good sign.

The 23rd Psalm—which I remember not from church but from a framed needlepoint eternally hanging in my grandmother's house—pops into my head: *Yea, though I walk through the valley of the shadow of death, I will fear no evil: for thou art with me; thy rod and thy staff they comfort me.* I think I finally get it— maybe. Rod, staff, and coffee: I'll take whatever comforts I can get.

At this moment I feel a dull ache in my abdomen on the left side, near the back of my ribcage. My upper-left back hurts from some tiny muscle I pulled during my thirty crunches. Weakened by cancer? My left armpit aches from Lumpy and surgery. An ache in my right hip, which has been coming and going for a year or so, is flaring up too. I feel broken down.

For a change of pace, Jenelle will accompany me to Dr. X's office this morning. She tells me she fears that Dr. X still won't have results; I fear that Dr. X will.

I walk out to the backyard. The day has dawned clear and cold. A mist rises from the golf course; the sun edges over the pine forest in the distance, bright orange and yellow, hopeful. It is a beautiful day for learning one's fate.

Kaily is awake. She and Jenelle are in a supportive mood. Kaily has made a paper hoop with yellow highlighter and black magic marker. It resembles a Livestrong bracelet and says, "Strong Like Gorilla!" So Kaily thinks of me as a big monkey. I slip on her bracelet and Jenelle begins to cry. Kaily cries, too. Cancer is the crying disease.

During the ride to the clinic, we do not speak of the impending news and arrive at the office of Dr. X at 9:28. CNN blares a repeating loop about the Bhutto assassination in Pakistan. I watch patiently. Moments later we are called over to pony up our co-pay prior to admittance. I have to show my ID first. ("No more life or death news for you, imposter!")

The nurse leads us to the exam room, checks my paperwork, and announces that we will go over the PET scan results.

"What about the CT scan?" I ask.

"There was a CT scan?" she says.

Jenelle and I exchange glances. "Yes," I say.

"Hmm... I'll check."

"Where's Dr. X?" I ask.

"Oh, she had to walk over to pathology for the report because nobody answered the phone over there. As usual."

I'd been imagining that Dr. X had been up late, poring over my reports, empty Starbucks cups strewn about, the scan results being committed to memory. She would then walk in, perfectly made up with a sexy doctor outfit and a plan in hand. It now occurs to me that Dr. X has read none of my paperwork since my last visit, and will be reviewing my case for the first time within the next few minutes, *if* she can find the reports in the pathology department. In the words of Kurt Vonnegut, so it goes.

At 9:48, still nothing. Jenelle reads reports from work. Our chamber has two chairs, a single stool on rollers and an exam table, all covered in ivory vinyl. The walls are unadorned; one is plum-colored and boasts a window. I open the blinds, revealing a parking lot and a freeway. People and patients walk by constantly, looking in. I close the blinds. The other three walls are lavender. By the door sits a gray trash can with a clear bag inside. There are no pictures hanging anywhere. The door is cream-colored, not quite matching the vinyl and definitely not matching the walls.

At 9:52, the nurse peeks in. "Dr. X is checking on something," she says and leaves.

Jenelle looks up, blinking as if struck on the temple by a pub dart. "I know what I'll do! I'll be your project manager!"

"The project to keep me alive?"

She usually doesn't like me to joke about my own mortality, but smiles this time. I accept her offer, because Jenelle is a superhuman organizer. Finally, at 9:55 Dr. X arrives, neither overtly made up nor sporting the Sexy Oncologist outfit I'd envisioned. Our eyes meet and there is a slight pause. I do not say anything, but she gets right to the point.

"You're not going to die of cancer," she says. I'm ready to bust out a big smile until she delivers her conclusion: "At least not from the cancer in your left axilla."

After Dr. X's announcement Jenelle looks relieved, but we are both engineers, and so the qualification doesn't go unnoticed. And here is another lesson that I have learned from my cancer experience (readers' experiences may vary): There is *never* definitive, clear-cut, unambiguous cancer news. There is *always* a catch.

We go over my PET scan, my CT scan, my recent blood work (wherein the doctors look for "markers" which are telltale signs of cancer), and a more in-depth pathology report which has been done on the original tissue removed by Doc Young.

"Other than your left axilla," Dr. X explains, "your CT scan and PET scan came up clean. There is no detectable cancer anywhere else. Your blood work and all affiliated markers came up normal."

Basically, I am healthy as a horse. (Except for Lumpy.) In my mind's movie, we break out into song, followed by a fade away. "And they lived happily ever after...." flashes upon the screen in lovely cursive font.

"There is, however," Dr. X says, "a slight change in your diagnosis. Based on the in-depth pathology report, you now have *Basaloid* Squamous Cell Carcinoma, Metastatic, Unknown Origin."

"What's with the 'basaloid?'" I ask.

"That's a variation on the squamous cell type," she says. "It shows up occasionally upon thorough review of pathology slides."

"So, what does that do to me?"

"It doesn't *do* anything to you, nor does it change the treatment options. It is a more precise definition of your cancer, but we look for it and treat it in the same manner."

Jenelle and I write feverishly.

"But back to the scan results," Dr. X continues. "The PET scan shows increased activity in the left axilla, measuring 1.8

centimeters in diameter."

This, she explains, is the remaining malignancy of which Doc Young spoke to Jenelle. It's the remainder of Lumpy that had us both crying in each other's arms the night of the biopsy surgery—the part that "doesn't look good."

"The CT scan shows the cancer area to be even larger," Dr. X says. "It measures 4.2 centimeters. However, this could be due to post-surgical swelling."

I do some mental math. At 2.54 centimeters per inch.... "What? That's freaking huge!"

"And one more thing," Dr. X says, "you also have an enlarged prostate."

"I have prostate cancer, too?"

"No, you have an enlarged prostate. Different cell type. However, we'll run some more blood work with PSA tests."

"So that's all?" I ask, sarcastically. "A growing mass in my armpit and I might not have prostate cancer?"

Dr. X nods noncommittally, then adds, "Well, not quite." She looks me in the eye. "We don't want you to have the 'Unknown Origin' label."

"Why not?" Jenelle says.

Dr. X looks over. "Trust me. We just don't."

"What does that mean, anyway?" Jenelle demands. "What is Unknown Origin?" *Yeah,* I think. *Good question.*

" For the moment, and until we learn more, you are officially classified as Unknown Origin, AKA Unknown Primary Origin, or Unknown Primary."

Dr. X elaborates as Jenelle and I continue to take notes. Unknown Origin does not imply, as it might seem upon initial inspection, that they do not know from whence I hail, nor is there confusion regarding species or alien beings. What it means is that the cancer named Lumpy did not originate in my left axilla; it metastasized from somewhere else. Lumpy's father is MIA. He's hiding or gone, or possibly too small to show up on a PET scan. He's a regular dead-beat dad.

I'm a big believer in cause and effect, and the thought that my cancer has spewed forth from an unknown spring is terrifying to say the least.

"It's not unheard of," Dr. X explains, sensing the growing tension in the room. "A small percentage of all cancer patients are classified as Unknown Origin." I ponder whether I find any comfort in that statement and cannot decide. "But," she continues. "We don't want you to be one of them."

Okay, now I have fully decided to *not* find comfort in being in the small percentage of Unknown Origin patients.

"So, here we are," I say. "What next?"

Dr. X will attempt to find Lumpy's old man. This requires more doctors and more tests. I am to visit (not necessarily in this order) a dermatologist, an Ear Nose and Throat doctor (ENT if you want to sound hip), and a gastroenterologist.

I listen patiently, but my skepticism is rampant. "What if these other doctors and tests still don't reveal the source cancer? Because, and correct me if I'm wrong here, if we don't know the source, then we don't know the cure."

"Correct," she confirms. "But relax. We have a mitigation strategy." She explains that as long as I remain in the Unknown Origin category, I will receive a PET scan every few months. *Forever....*

PET scans until death-do-us-part sounds better than just death, but I am a closure kind of guy. On an intellectual level, I am on board and ready to sign up. On an emotional level, I am untrusting and wary. I feel that this "mitigation strategy" is an ambiguous non-answer. Lumpy's pappy will keep hiding out in the dark alleys and cheap motels of my innards, humping like mad and producing offspring that are larger, faster and ever more aggressive.

I politely ask Dr. X about getting Lumpy the hell out of my body ASAP. I feel like asking, *Can we do it here in the office, right now?*, but resist the urge. The course of action, she tells me, will involve chemotherapy and radiation. But first more testing. Jenelle and I ask approximately 175 more questions, but in the end learn little else. We leave.

How do I feel? Pretty damned well, but, as they say, it ain't over, not by a long shot. Still ahead are tests, exams, and then radiation and chemotherapy. I feel somehow better off than Lance when he was diagnosed (after all, I am not riddled with tumors), and look at him now! I pep up and the mood going home is light; even Jenelle appears more upbeat.

After we arrive home, I dumbly decide to Google the odds of survival for people diagnosed with basaloid squamous-cell carcinoma, or BSCC in medical shorthand. I type "BSCC" into the search box, along with "metastatic" and "unknown origin." Click, click. Pause. *Oh, shit.* People with this combination die soon, and often. Can I actually die more than once? It does not matter, for I am a dead man regardless.

I do not tell Jenelle of my Web discovery; instead I traverse the phone system and leave a panicky message for Dr. X to call me. Two hours later, she actually does. I explain what I've read on the Internet.

"First off," she says sternly, "don't do that. Don't surf the net looking for your prognosis because it will scare you. Second, a simple reading of statistics is misleading. Included in those numbers are old people, smokers, old smokers, and people with other health problems. I stick to my original statement. You *will not* die from this."

"But I could die later, if the Unknown Origin makes a screaming comeback," I say.

"True," she admits, "and you could be killed by a bus tomorrow. Let's worry about one thing at a time and treat what we know about *now*."

I hang up and come away a little calmer. I lay face up on the floor in the middle of my office and close my eyes. The two and a half weeks between Dr. Young's scalpel and today's PET scan results have been a war of attrition upon my nerves and very soul. I have attempted to be serene and strong and accepting, even of imminent death, should that be my fate, but the gas tank is now on "E." I want to be John Wayne right now, or Lance Armstrong, ready to fight the good fight. But I feel scared, depressed and most of all tired. I can't allow myself to fall asleep, though—there are more appointments.

The ENT

I am supposed to see both the ENT and gastroenterologist today, but Jenelle accidentally multi-tasked me out of that plan by scheduling the appointments too closely together. So I end up cancelling the colon-meister. We are cancer novices, after all. I do manage to make my ENT visit, though. He is in the same medical complex as the cancer center, but on a different floor. I do not have an ENT of my own, so Dr. X recommended Dr. Uvula.

Doc Uvula has a computer station set up for enrolling new patients. There, I enter my life history, medical history, insurance information, and driver's license number. Upon completion, I wait with Jenelle in the waiting room, which is pleasantly less crowded than the other ones I've been frequenting lately. The whole building is fairly new and nice.

Doctor Uvula has piercing eyes, as though he's taking in my life—odd drinking stories and all—through my pupils, and does not find it to be all that enthralling. He is sincere and pleasant, answering questions in a calm way devoid of condescension. He then sends Jenelle to the waiting room and squirts some of the nastiest-tasting goo ever made into my nostrils in preparation for "the scoping." I gag and nearly spit it back out upon his pristine white coat.

Next, I sit before a cart containing a video monitor and a flexible mini-snake James Bond camera with which Doc U looks down people's throats and up into their sinuses. I find it less than soothing to feel a mini camera snuck up my right nostril and on toward my brain, and then downright distressing to see what it sees on the video monitor. As visually unappealing as sinuses are, they are less offensive than the view down the throat. Doc U has me close my mouth, hold my nose and give a good push from the lungs. The vista toward the vocal cords at this point looks amazingly like the alien in "Predator." Dr. Uvula immediately gives me a clean bill of health. "There is no cancer visible," he says.

"What about cancer that's not visible?"

I detect a bit of impatience clouding Doc U's serene countenance. Maybe he's not used to people asking questions; I should have warned him that I am an engineer.

"As I said, you're cancer-free in these regions."

"Are you sure?"

"Look, I just told you..." he sighs. I've done it; I've gotten to the man. I didn't mean to, but there it is. "You don't have cancer in any of the areas I've examined." He speaks sternly, with authority.

Rather than being offended or hurt, I am ecstatic. "Right on, Doc!"

I still have a nasty taste in my mouth, but now it is the taste of joy. I tell Jenelle the news and she is happy. For now. But by the time I get home the joy has faded as I still must face the Colonel of Colon tomorrow. I do myself a favor and stay off of Google.

The Gastroenterologist

After a good night's sleep, I begin to grow fond of the idea that I could be around for a while. But I worry about the Unknown Origin cancer that is as yet undetected and therefore untreated. I want it gone, and Lumpy gone with it. Regarding Lumpy, Dr. X recommends radiation as the primary treatment, with a side order of "light" chemotherapy (same great taste, but less destructive to my healthy bits). The light chemo is not the primary treatment, but is intended to weaken Lumpy so that the radiation will kill him while he isn't looking. I latch onto the dead-Lumpy idea to the point of a high-school crush. I picture a Cookie-like funeral, but then immediately abandon that idea as too good for the bastard. I'd just as soon see him explode via a thermonuclear device shoved up where the Lumpy sun don't shine.

Jenelle and I arrive at the office of Doc Wherethesundon'tshine. I've never met the man; he is another recommendation of Dr. X's. His office is in a medical building near the local mall. The waiting room is full, with only two seats open. I expected the walls to be either pink or the color of shit, but instead they are gray; the carpet is a dark pepper. The seats are covered in black leather and turn out to be *the* comfiest waiting room chairs anywhere (a good sign, especially given the subject matter).

I journal; Jenelle reads. I am called up front to fill out the usual paperwork. I dream of a universal form that I could fill out once and give in photocopy form to all doctors. This is because all doctors ask for the same information, and I am sick of providing it.

We get called into the back and meet the Doc. He is a small man with a gentle handshake, and has soft hands—exceptionally soft. In fact, I find myself wanting to hold one of his little hands and one of Jenelle's at the same time for comparison, but resist the urge. I ponder the softness and size of his digits a brief moment and decide that these are both highly desirable qualities in a gastroenterologist. I am in the right place.

Doc W explains the procedures, which for the dear reader's sake I will not cover in great detail; basically, he will scope me from both ends. I feel the urge to break out into song: "You take the high road and I'll take the low road, and I'll be in David's esophagus a 'fore ye!" I wisely resist the urge.

"You will be under for the whole procedure." I find this idea reassuring. Doc W then prescribes a colonoscopy make-ready kit, which I am surprised to learn can be purchased in any local pharmacy. "Any questions?"

"Yes. How soon can we do this?"

He looks up his calendar on the computer and schedules me for Monday at the hospital adjacent to the cancer center. "Is that soon enough?" he says.

I nod, then I'm sent to pay and receive further instructions. Monday is New Year's Eve.

The nurse gives me a sheet of instructions (no coffee; clear liquids only, nothing at all after midnight). She tells me that I will receive results two weeks after the exam.

"Two weeks!" I exclaim.

Doc W catches my eye. "Relax," he says, "I will take care of you." He then tells me that he will inform Jenelle of the results right after the procedure, while I regain consciousness (assuming, of course, that I regain consciousness).

I arrive home and test the range of motion of my left arm: seventy-five percent. Not bad. This makes me think that I should make it back to taekwondo soon. Maybe without all the pushups, but soon.

The Dermatologist

In the afternoon, Jenelle and I make one more trip, to the dermatologist. I've had a history of sun-related skin damage since college in the early '80s. I am as white as they come, an Irish/Scotch blend back through various generations of freckle-faced individuals. This means I am always on the losing side of a daily battle with the Texas sun. The Spanish vernacular for my complexion translates to "bucket of milk."

Basal cells are brought on by sun damage, and there is also a type of skin cancer called squamous-cell skin cancer. It might be a stretch, but based on cell type alone there could be a skin-cancer connection with Lumpy. It is not a wholly unreasonable trail to follow into the dark territory of the Unknown Origin.

In order to follow up on all of this, I must go to a new dermatologist. The one I used to see has retired since my last visit, a few months back. Dr. X recommends Dr. Skin, a dermatologist with quite a name about town. His office is cleverly hidden, tucked off a side road near a large medical establishment on the north end of town. I motor past his driveway twice before spotting it.

Doc Skin's parking lot is full, and the waiting room is packed. But the waiting room is quite nice, like a den in a large home. It has quality periodicals (a poetry journal, architectural magazines), and homey incandescent lamps. There are windows everywhere looking out upon green tropical gardens. Notably absent is a giant-screen, blaring television. I fill out yet another set of forms, and it is upon completion of same that I realize that our insurance company will not pay for this particular doctor (because it is stated as such on his form in bold-face font). Not ideal, but here I am.

In the exam room, there hangs a Ralph Steadman print, signed, along with two nice Audubon-style bird prints, plus a number of high-quality photos. Jenelle spies an issue of "The American Scholar" and picks it up. I find an older issue of same, filled with essays. Doc Skin comes in wearing a bowtie. He looks a bit like post-*Deliverance* Ned Beatty. I tell my story and Doc Skin asks a lot of questions. He seems to find my case intriguing, and while I talk he examines my skin for basal and squamous cells. The whole scene reminds me of monkeys grooming.

Doc Skin points out a couple of spots that might need attention (nothing urgent), and then explains that he thinks Dr. X could be right; there could be a skin-cancer connection at play here. I explain that my previous dermatologist has retired. He asks the name, and I tell him: Dr. Gone. Doc Skin knows Dr. Gone personally. He requests that I get all of my old files from Dr. Gone, the sooner the better. The more Doc Skin preens and hears of my story, the more excited he becomes, and I picture some serious feces chucking in our immediate future. He says he'll call me once he reviews my files.

$95 later, we go home. My follow-up visit with Dr. X is Thursday. But before that, I have a follow up with my surgeon, Doc Young.

December 30

I work out, spending twenty minutes on the escalator machine at level eleven. I do twenty-five slow pushups on my knees without much discomfort in the shoulder. I work the legs and stretch. As a reward afterward, I go to the mega-grocery store near home and buy colonoscopy supplies: a pair of pills and a "kit" containing a plastic jug and some foil packets of flavored diarrhea crystals. It all appears benign enough, almost like it could be fun.

I arrive at home, take the two pills and go about my business. Diarrhea commences shortly thereafter. Next comes the jug: I have a choice between lemon-lime or cherry-orange powder (no berry delicious). I pick lemon-lime, fill the jug to the line with water and dump the pouch in. At the appropriate time I chugalug. I wait.

Knock, knock. Who's there? Shit, and lots of it! Mr. David, meet Mr. Toilet. As soon as I leave Mr. Toilet, I miss him badly and sprint back for more bonding. I try to sneak off again, but he calls before I get to the door. I violate laws of physics by shitting more than I weigh. At halftime I am allowed to "eat" some chicken broth (comes right back out) and some Jell-O (comes right back out). You ask: Dave, just how much watery shit can one human produce in an evening? Answer: 11,000 gallons. And does that ever make me *hungry*! But there will be no food or water after midnight (not that it would stay), and none in the morning until after I get home from The Probing.

In an abrupt turnaround from the Christmas Eve Scotch-induced warm fuzzy feelings I had for 2007, now I feel genuinely sick about it. Just before bed, I have a memory dating back to 1982: I had a high school classmate who went to get his wisdom teeth out, and opted for general anesthesia. He never woke up. I've gone twenty-five years without that memory, but here it is, clear as my last trip to Mr. Toilet. I decide that if I die from the anesthesia, it will save me from having to go through cancer treatment, but then again, I might die with a probe up my ass. Decisions, decisions.

New Year's Eve

I awaken, and with the time freed up by my inability to eat or drink anything, head straight for the journal:

Today is The Scoping. I shit out the last of 2007 over the course of a dozen-plus trips to the bathroom yesterday, until about 11:30 PM. I continue to chafe at the lack of treatment for cancer—I've had none yet, however, the logical half of my brain allows that the tests are necessary and could help me in the long run. The Cowboys were annihilated—beaten like a cur dog and generally made to look like ass. Not a good end of the season. They can reflect during bye week.

We show up at the hospital; I don the gown and lie down on a gurney to be wheeled into The Probery. I bid Jenelle adieu until my ass is re-covered in recovery. I am hooked up to a heart monitor and before you know it, here comes the anesthesiologist. Will he be Dr. Happy or Dr. Death? My guess is that I will not care once I am doped up.

The vein is struck (without compliments); the drugs enter. I feel a brief rush of euphoria, and laugh at how hilarious the probe looks before waking up, all finished. My ass is a bit sore, but I can't tell if it's from The Probing, too much rough toilet paper from the prior day, or perhaps some sort of Abu Ghraib tom-foolery with digital cameras and people grinning while giving the "thumbs up." Mental note: check YouTube.

Doc Wherethesundon'tshine tells Jenelle that I'm all clear; no signs of cancer in either end, or at any point in between. She informs me of this while I lay in recovery. This is a huge relief. But there *is* something—isn't there always? Doc W comes in and explains that there is a bit of light scarring where the esophagus attaches to the stomach—possible acid reflux.

"Nothing to worry about," he says.

"But acid reflux is a problem for stressed-out people! I'm a calm person!"

"Yes," he smiles, "and I have a fifteen-inch pecker." He doesn't really say this, but he does scoff at my assertions of being a calm person.

New Year's Day

With no debut on YouTube and most of the soreness already gone, I work out. I set the escalator stair machine on twelve for twenty minutes, do a full-blown leg workout with post-workout stretching, and manage twenty-five proper pushups in good form (not on my knees). If I can keep people from cutting on me, I hope to work it back up to fifty, just like the good old days. I still don't have a full range of motion in my left shoulder, but it is close enough for government work. All of this returning strength pleases me and gives me optimism. I feel clean. From the inside.

4 CHOOSING A TREATMENT CENTER

I do a bit of non-scary Internet research regarding the Big C and its human side. It is not scary because I am not reading about BSCC. It turns out that many cancer victims (survivors, sufferers, reveling bacchanalians—however we decide to think of ourselves) feel compelled to remember cancer anniversaries. I theorize that this is so we can celebrate if we make it to Year One without a recurrence, or at all. But fixing my cancer anniversary is a puzzle; I felt Lumpy way back in the summer but wasn't diagnosed until December. I decide upon December 17 as my anniversary because this was the date when I first heard the news, officially, from Doc Young. I try to picture myself on my first cancer anniversary, but then decide against it just in case (curse of the Cyclops and all that).

The girls and Jenelle are greatly calmed by all of the cancer-free zones that have been staked out around my body. That, and all my exercising give them the illusion that I'm in total control. Calmness reigns. Except in my own head. I need some comfort food.

* * *

Cars are my comfort food. They are Jack in the Box tacos for my escapist brain cells. I have a lot of those cells and always have; nowadays they are threatening to take over. I look at cars, read about them (I have multiple car magazine subscriptions, but many are in Jenelle's name so they're not really mine, are they?), talk about them, lust after them, buy them, sell them, and drive the crap out of them. Even the lame ones.

Looking at cars on Craig's List becomes a nifty little escape from reality, and so does thinking about actually buying one. I find out about a former boss selling his late '80s Mustang GT convertible, complete with hideous body cladding and pimped-out louvered taillights. The styling of this car is so awful that the passage of time has made it cool. I call him up and get a price. Once I hear a dollar figure I realize that I ought to watch my money now, because Lumpy is liable to eat it all. My former boss gets to keep his Mustang.

The near-miss prompts me to consider selling Little Blue to raise cancer money—but that would be crazy! Little Blue is my BMW M Roadster (think Mazda Miata on steroids and Red Bull), and also my favorite car ever—I could never sell her. However, I do feel slightly conflicted over keeping her: one theory is that Lumpy could be the offspring of skin cancer, which is exacerbated by sunlight, therefore maybe I shouldn't own a convertible. It turns out that I should probably not even own a car, as high speed has become a place I like to visit often. Risky behavior is feeling less so.

Meanwhile, back at the ranch, I begin a new job. My one-man consulting firm has been doing well enough, keeping me mellow for two and a half years, but upon cancer diagnosis I finally figure out that there is a gaping hole in my business plan: If I do not work, I do not get paid. If I do not get out and sell my consulting services, I do not work. If I get sick, I can do neither. I need benefits.

Firm D has been my primary client for the past eight months or so. They like me and vice versa. Firm D makes me a handsome employment offer. In addition to craving benefits, I am a bit of a harlot when it comes to my engineering career path, and so can be bought if the price is right.

Firm D is similar to my own firm, but with ten years more experience under its belt. If I sign on, I'll report directly to the two owners, with whom I get along quite well. I'll continue doing the same high-end work, but exclusively for them, and in their building. The only downsides to this scenario are a commute (ten miles as the crow flies from my house) and regular office hours.

In the course of deciding whether to accept Firm D's offer, I meet with the owners and tell them about my cancer. I explain that if they want to rescind I will understand, as they will be buying defective merchandise. This conversation takes place after my first visit with Dr. X, but before I know the PET scan results, so I don't know if I will soon become too sick to work.

The owners of Firm D listen patiently. I repeat my offer to bow out.

One of the owners looks me in the eye and says, "The offer stands."

"But what if I get sick?"

"The offer stands."

How's that for refreshing? Now I work at Firm D. The salient point here is this: Firm D now provides me with health insurance, sick days, vacation days, and a base salary. So cancer's bad timing isn't all bad. Hooking up with Firm D turns out to be a stroke of good luck, providing me with some security during the cancer-fest.

* * *

I have developed a theory about stress; I call it the Bucket Theory. Each human has the capacity to absorb a certain amount of stress without freaking out. This capacity is The Bucket. Whether the Bucket is ten percent full or ninety percent full doesn't matter, because so long as it does not overflow, calm will reign. If my Bucket is fifty percent full, I can absorb another forty-nine percent and still remain calm. However, once the bucket is, say, ninety-nine percent full, a mere two-percent dollop of stress can come along and unleash the furies of hell, as the Bucket will then be overflowing. Once stress has gone over the top, that sucker keeps overflowing with every new incident of tension until I can find a place of quiet dignity to empty it down and restore balance.

Following this line of reasoning, it behooves me to keep my Bucket's stress level as low as possible on a daily basis. Why? Because shit happens, and often in quantities representing significant percentages of Bucket fill. If I keep the daily level low, I can absorb a pretty good hit and still remain calm. If I am constantly running at ninety percent, a couple of minor events (road rudeness, long checkout line at the grocery store) can set the stage for a nuclear meltdown when I get home only to learn that Bonehead has dug up a shrub and I have foolishly shrunk Jenelle's bras in the dryer (again). You can do the math.

So, here is the kicker: Cancer tends to keep the Bucket topped up, or darn near the top. Combine that with indecision over treatment options, add a new job, and there is trouble in paradise.

* * *

The idea of income and benefits security calms me as I embark on my first commute in two and a half years. It is January second, and I arrive at a building to work with other humans. I show up in time for Firm D's 9:00 AM meeting. Within moments I am informed that my project is already late. We are swamped; the schedule is tight. After the meeting, I find that I must share an office with two other men, Armchair and Danny Dell, our IT guy. I had been hoping for privacy, as having cancer entails a lot of telephone calls (doctors, loved ones, friends to vent upon, more doctors, insurance companies, and more doctors).

I take a seat at my new desk and make small talk, trying act like all is well (no cancer going on here, boys!), but soon find that sharing an office, and especially a phone, makes this impossible. I spill the beans and tell my suite-mates all about my cancer. Armchair and Danny Dell hardly know me; now they know I have cancer. I actually feel a bit less stressed after telling them and warning them about cancer-related phone calls.

"Are you going to MD Anderson?" Armchair says.

"I haven't decided."

"You're a fool if you don't go to MD Anderson. You have to go to MD Anderson!"

"Have you ever had cancer?"

"No."

"Anyone close to you?"

"Not in the last couple of decades. But you have to go to MD Anderson!"

As time passes, I receive additional unsolicited feedback from

Jenelle's mother Jo and brother Jimmy; also from my own Mom and Dad, and many others. There's a theme: *You're a fool if you don't go to MD Anderson. You have to go to MD Anderson.*

It turns out that I have an acquaintance who is supposed to be my "in" at MD Anderson. It's always about who you know, even in the cancer biz. As it turns out, this "in" suggests that I go and punch my information into the MD Anderson web site. It occurs to me that anybody could do this, even without an "in." I punch my data on the Saturday before my first day of work at Firm D. In auto-reply, the MD Anderson web site assures me that I will be contacted post haste.

I wait for a reply until my first day at Firm D. Nothing; *nada.* No direct emails from humans and no call backs. I find a phone number on the computer-generated email that thanked me for punching in. I call from my desk at Firm D.

This call plunges me into the labyrinthine hell of the MD Anderson phone system. I am bounced from flunkie to flunkie, department to department. I give my last name to each operator:

"Baskett," I say.

"Vasquez?"

"No, Baskett."

"Gasket?"

"No, Baskett, like Basketball."

"B-A-S-K-E-T-B-A-L-L?"

"No, *like* basketball, not actually basketball."

The MD Anderson phone system hangs up on me several times during various internal transfers. I begin to take it personally. Each time I call back, I have to navigate a computer phone menu system until a human comes on. Then I must repeat my name, my diagnosis, and its location.

"Left axilla," I say.

"Left what?"

"Axilla."

"I'm sorry, what?"

"Left armpit!"

"Ooh, I don't like the sound of that!"

"Yeah, how do you think I feel?"

I spell my name. Again. I get hung up on. Again. I keep calling and finally get through to a human who transfers me to what she assures me is the correct department. Yet another human answers. The woman asks what cancer I have and where I have it. I repeat my story.

"What?" she says. "We don't treat that. Why did you call this department?"

I hold the receiver in front of my face and stare at it a moment. Will it really do any good to slam it against the top of the desk until it breaks? I put it back to my ear.

"I'm not the one who called this department, I was transferred by one of you MD Anderson people!"

"Hold on, let me transfer you." Click. A dial tone vibrates my skull.

I wade through the menu once again and get connected to the person who just told me I called the wrong department.

"Mr. Basketball?" she says.

"Yes, that's me."

"I'm starting to recognize your voice. How can I help you?"

Her mind seems to have been wiped clean of the previous conversation—rebooted, as it were. I take advantage of the situation and plead my case. She becomes so confused that she transfers me to her supervisor, who transfers me to a human of functional intelligence. Her name is Ms. Helpful.

I converse with Ms. Helpful and find that I am finally getting somewhere.

"When can I get an appointment?" I say.

"Not until we enter you into the system."

"Then let's enter me into the system."

"You need to have your pathology report and any other medical reports sent over ASAP. These will be evaluated, and the correct doctor notified."

"Okay. How do I get my reports?"

"Go ask for them."

"But you never answered my question. Can you enter me into the system?"

"No. Not yet. We can't enter you into the system without a pathology report."

"Then I get an appointment?"

"You can't have an appointment until we enter you into the system."

Is this a Catch-22? I'm not sure, but it sure is pissing me off, even though Ms. Helpful is making an effort.

All the while that I battle the MD Anderson phone system, and it is a long while—first day at the new job, mind you—another engineer and my boss keep coming in and asking my office mates for drawings and information and whatnot. They occasionally ask me engineering questions as well. So I am trying to work, trying to wade through phone hell, and trying not to go insane all at the same time. In the meantime, Basaloid Squamous Lumpy is growing larger and stronger inside my body, laughing evilly all the while I do not receive treatment.

Comes 3:30. I recall from an earlier stint at a large corporation in Houston that this is the onset of rush hour. If I leave much later, I will be stuck in traffic for God knows how long, time I feel that I cannot spare because I have more cancer phone calls to make from the house. However, I feel badly for leaving early after arriving here late, even though I have an agreement with the owners of Firm D that I can work from home as needed.

I vacillate and argue with the voices in my head, finally deciding to leave at 3:30. This stresses me out, as traffic is already thick. I arrive home and check messages but no medical rescuers have called back. Trying to call Dr. X, I reach only phone menus, and hang up.

I call Jenelle and sound, even to myself, like a madman. Relax, she says. One of Jenelle's great fears in life is being licked by a cockroach. I tell her to imagine one squirming around inside her left armpit, one that can kill her. She gives me the classic, "There, there." I feel a modicum of concern from her, but little in the way of empathy. How can she feel empathy unless I manage to place a deadly, licking cockroach into her left armpit? How will I do that? While she sleeps, maybe?

It's not her fault, I tell myself. In any event, she does not share my urgency and speaks in placating tones, as one might to a child who has dropped his already peeled banana. I feel worse after calling Jenelle. I want to call Dr. X again, but find myself paralyzed. I feel lonely, helpless, and scared, like I am the only person on earth with cancer. I am not just in a rush; I am becoming neurotic, psychotic, and obsessive. It feels like I'm going to explode.

I call Dr. X and leave a message on the nurse's answering machine: "Please call me back!" It is 4:15 PM, well past the daily deadline. By 5:30 there's been no call back. I lay on the floor of my home office, face down. I say the Alcoholics Anonymous Serenity Prayer several times, even though I am not a member. I probably should be.

"God, grant me the serenity to accept the things I cannot change, the courage to change the things I can, and the wisdom to know the difference."

I wait. Nothing. I say it again. I do not feel that I have been granted the wisdom to know the difference. What I feel is carpet pressing into my forehead.

Jenelle calls back to check on me, but I am inconsolable, even though she is being quite nice, with her tone now approaching empathy. By now I do not want to talk with her or anybody else who cannot irradiate me or inject me with chemotherapy drugs on the spot.

I flip over and stare at the ceiling. *I am a fool if I do not go to MD Anderson.* I am a fool who cannot even freaking talk to a damned MD Anderson doctor due to an admissions Catch-22. I am between a rock and a hard medical bureaucracy. What if I start treatment at the local cancer center instead? Will that kill me? Is there no recourse but MD Anderson? Armchair says so.

But for me there is a catch: MD Anderson treated my father-in-law Jim, and now he is dead. They are zero for one on my scorecard. But if I do not go there I'm an idiot. Only a *fool* would not go there. But I cannot get in there, at least not fast enough for my taste. And if I get in tomorrow, which I will not, then who knows how long until treatment begins, and I want cancer the hell out of my body right now, right this second!

I reach up and feel under my arm. I feel the scar over the lump.

Lumpy is growing. He likes it there in the axilla, giving off dull aches of contentment, sparking stress and numbness down my arm, like fire ants venturing forth awaiting the bite signal, to further metastasize into other organs and lymph nodes. He grows with impunity, fertilized by the very stress he causes. He is the devil.

If I stick with Dr. X, my treatment begins at the end of this week or the beginning of next week at the latest. But that will be the wrong decision, according to all of the non-cancer experts who have not been through what I have been through, seen the doctors I have seen, or undergone the tests that I have undergone. At 5:50 PM my cell phone rings. It is Ms. Helpful from MD Anderson. She takes my information over the phone to put me into the system, taking my word that I will soon come up with a pathology report. I am now in the system! The other line beeps. I switch over; it is Dr. X's nurse. I tell her I want the pathology report sent to MD Anderson.

"Which pathology report?"

"The only one," I say. "The detailed one that Dr. X authorized."

This does not seem to make sense to the nurse. I ask her if I can call her back, as I am on the other line. She explains that I cannot because the phones are a one-way automated system—there is no way for me to call in except to leave a message. I switch over and ask Ms. Helpful from MD Anderson if I can call her right back. She explains that I cannot because they use a one-way automated system, and that I will have to leave a message. I am stuck.

Dr. X's nurse offers to call me back in a few minutes, thus breaking the stalemate. I accept. I ask Ms. Helpful a lot of questions, centered around how long it will take to get my initial evaluation appointment at MDA. She tells me that if she had all the required paperwork sitting in her hand (which she does not), and if a doctor had already reviewed it (obviously impossible), they could see me in twenty days.

"Twenty days?" I ask. Lumpy giggles meanly.

"Yes," she says. "Twenty days."

Cancer R Us, Cancer Warehouse, Cancer Depot... where is the quick fix, the drop-in solution? It's crunch time, and I seem to be in line at the DMV of cancer. Beep! It is Dr. X's nurse calling me back while I am still speaking with Ms. Helpful from MDA. She has figured out that there is, in fact, a pathology report somewhere, but cannot put her hands on it until tomorrow. Another day burnt. Lumpy guffaws and grows a few more mutant cells for good measure.

I hang up with everybody. I won't know squat until I get my reports to MDA. They are starting my case in the "Head and Neck" department. Is that the right place? Nobody knows.

My Bucket runneth over.

January 3

On my second day of employment with Firm D, I manage not to make it in to work. Instead I take a sick day and go to my follow-up with Doc Young. I am running late because of traffic and full parking lots. The line to the elevators is long. I'll show them all—I'll run up the stairs. I am strong! I'm an athlete!

I run five floors and arrive horribly winded; I might puke. People stare with pity while I lean over holding onto my knees. Look at the poor sickly patient with lung trouble.

I catch my breath while Doc Young fires up the monitor in my exam room. Here are all of my test results, pathology reports, blood work results, the whole nine yards, all in his system. He is *the* most organized doctor I have ever run across. He checks under my arm and tells me that the wound is healing well.

"Great! Now when will it quit looking like a pair of sewn-together...uhm, when will the scar go down, I mean?"

"Soon," he says.

I tell him my whole story, pretty much all that has transpired since our last visit together. I tell him that I am scared and don't know what to do; don't know whether to stay here at the local cancer hospital or go to MD Anderson. He listens patiently.

"If you had a more common case..." he says.

"Garden variety?" I say, interrupting.

He chuckles. "Yeah, garden variety. Then the treatment protocols are all well established and it pretty much doesn't matter where you get treated, within reason. But in your case, that unknown primary is a bitch. It certainly is within your rights as a patient, and not unreasonable, to seek more opinions."

"But what would *you* do, Doc?"

"Dude, I'd get treated right here. I'd have them treat what we know about and worry about finding the unknown primary as we go. Parallel path, you know what I mean?"

Logic works well with me sometimes, but I am way out of my comfort zone when it comes to medicine and cancer. A big fluffy cloud of uncertainty continues to float between my ears.

"So, why wouldn't I just go to MD Anderson?"

"In my opinion, time. It takes time to get into their queue to see if they'll even accept you, then time to get you scheduled into their system; time to get re-examined and re-evaluated. They might start from scratch and re-do all of your tests and scans."

"Why the hell would they do that?"

"It's just how they work. And after all that, your treatment would probably be the same as it would here."

"Shit, this is a big freaking choice...it's not like Ford versus Chevy—this could have dire consequences. I tell you Doc, I keep feeling pressure to go to MD Anderson. But if I wait and do that, you say that a lot of time will pass—time I don't want to waste. I want freaking treatment, and I want it right freaking now."

"Hey, like I said, I'd get treatment here. You may not have met Dr. The Man yet, but he runs this whole hospital, and he is The Man. He's famous in the world of radiation oncology, and radiation is your primary treatment, so..."

"So stay?"

"So I'm saying it's up to you, man, but you know what I would do if it were me."

"I'll think about it."

There remains one more topic: Doc Young says he may be required to do one more surgery on me: a "portacath." This is a plastic valve inserted just under the skin near the sternum, and is used to administer chemotherapy. One end of the portacath accepts the chemicals, and the other end is attached semi-permanently (until surgically removed) to a vein. "It's no big deal, man," he says, "I do them all the time." I ponder a plastic conduit to a vein sewn beneath my skin. A shudder ensues, followed by visions of mainlining whiskey through it. "You might not need one," he says. "It's up to Dr. X. But if you do, it's no big deal." I have read about portacaths in Lance's book, and cannot work up any excitement about them.

Just before leaving it occurs to me to ask the obvious: "Dr. Young, would it be possible for you to print out a copy off all my reports?"

He reaches around to the computer keyboard, manipulates the mouse a couple of times and clicks. "Done," he says.

It was that easy. I pick up the reports on my way out.

Confronting Dr. X

I go home for a while and stare at my office ceiling, unable to make up my mind. What I can do, I realize, is scan all my reports and email them to Ms. Helpful at MD Anderson. This provides a good deal of relief.

Jenelle shows up and I tell her about what Doc Young said. She doesn't know what to do either. We have to leave anyway, for an appointment with Dr. X.

Back at the cancer center, ID is checked, co-pay is collected; cable news blares. Dr. X reviews the follow-up test results and doctor visits I've had thus far. In a nutshell, this is what we discuss:

ENT: Clear.

Doc Wherethesundon'tshine: Clear.

Dermatologist: Good theory, but an unclear connection. At any rate, not a hindrance to the treatment protocol.

"What about my blood work for the PSA level? Do I also have prostate cancer?"

She flips through her paperwork. "Point six three."

Jenelle and I stare at her. "Okay," I venture, "let me re-phrase that. Do I also have prostate cancer?"

"Point six three is good, as in no cancer. The healthy range is zero to four."

This is a much greater relief than I had anticipated—must be an anatomical proximity thing.

Dr. X reviews and summarizes Where We Are At: Lumpy remains a thriving entity. No other cancer has been detected, so I still have the dreaded "unknown origin" label. What To Do: Treat Lumpy with chemotherapy and radiation, followed by PET scans and close monitoring for however long I care to live thereafter. Dr. X tells us that she is confident she can "kill" the cancer under my arm, no problem.

"Are you sure?" I say, reflexively.

"Look," she says. "Nothing can survive radiation."

"Does that include me?"

"I meant cancer cells."

Jenelle and I look at each other. Jim did not survive radiation; his lungs were dysfunctionally inflamed after his last treatment, and he had to use an oxygen bottle until the end. His cancer did not get killed, but he sure did. Jenelle must be thinking what I am thinking because she brings up small-cell lung cancer.

"You don't have small-cell lung cancer," Dr. X says to me. "Your radiation will not affect your lungs." She recommends two doses of chemo, but will re-evaluate as things go along.

"And that will work?" Jenelle says.

"Yes," Dr. X says. She turns to me. "You can emerge cancer-free after treatment."

Jenelle takes some notes and she and I look at each other again. There comes an awkward silence.

"So," Dr. X says, "are you ready to begin treatment?"

"Yes," I say, because I like Dr. X. I trust Dr. X. But I feel forced to confront Dr. X. "Look," I add, "This sounds good, like you have it under control, and I find you to be a competent doctor." I pause to gather more words.

"Oh, gosh," she says, "I feel a lot better about myself now. I'm competent!"

Jenelle gets a big laugh off of that one.

"Yeah, well," I say, "sorry, but you know what I mean. Anyway, the thing is, I'm feeling a lot of pressure to go to MD Anderson."

Dr. X frowns upon this idea, literally. She also shakes her head. "I don't think MD Anderson is such a good idea."

"But friends call and tell me I need to go there; Jenelle's mother tells me the same thing, even though her husband went there and died. Also, Jenelle's brother tells me to go there. And my parents and people I'm barely acquainted with are pressuring me to go to MD Anderson. A guy at the office who doesn't even know me tells me I'm a fool if I don't go there. The place is freaking world famous! So it's a bit of a tough sell for me to use our local cancer center."

Dr. X gazes at me curiously, as though she has discovered a new species of monkey. I think she will become angry, but she remains placid.

"Listen," she says, "you are free to do what you please. I understand this perspective, and it *is* tough for us to compete with the marketing of MD Anderson. They're the Home Depot of cancer hospitals."

"Hey, that's what I thought!"

"Yes, they're Home Depot, and we're just the corner hardware shop."

"If it was just a matter of hardware," I say, "then I actually like the corner store for better service. But this... this could be life or death."

"You're not going to die from this—assuming we get on with treatment."

"But the unknown origin!" Jenelle says.

"Look," Dr. X says, "squamous cells occur in the following places: Lung, skin, upper GI, anus, and head and neck, which means the mouth and throat. We've screened and scanned each place visually, with a CT scan and with a PET scan. We cannot find the origin, true enough, but neither will MD Anderson."

"In your opinion," Jenelle says.

"Yes, in my opinion."

There comes a pause. "Can you," I say, "I mean *would* you please tell me something that will keep me here? I like this place and your practice, but I'm on a razor's edge. Please throw me a bone here."

"Okay," replies Dr. X, beginning to look enthused. "Number one: This place is owned and operated by Dr. The Man. He is practically world renowned in the field of radio oncology. He has developed a radiation treatment for prostate cancer that is, literally, now being taught for use around the world. Your primary treatment will be radiation with chemo to enhance that primary treatment. If *I* had to receive radiation, I'd want to receive it from Dr. The Man.

"Number two: MD Anderson is a money machine. They have mind-boggling cash flow, and with that comes a mind-boggling advertising budget. People have heard of them, to be fair, because they *are* good, but also because they advertise often and everywhere—all over the world, in fact. However, if you still want MD Anderson to look at you, you won't hurt my feelings in the slightest. The choice is yours."

I breathe in and try to make sense of all of this. "Okay, so now we know what I have and mostly where I have it. I understand from talking to Dr. Young that there will be a delay before I could be looked at by MD Anderson."

"True," she says, "and did he also tell you that MD Anderson will re-do all of the tests and exams that you've already undergone?"

"He said they might."

"They *will* re-do everything," she says, "I've seen it myself. Also, they will enroll you in a clinical study, because that's what they do. Here we use what is called the standard treatment protocol, which is what MDA should give you, except that they won't because you'll be in some sort of clinical study."

"Okay," I say, "they'll re-do everything."

"Yes," she says.

"I added it up," I say, "and it seems like all this MD Anderson delay could be another month—"

"Or more," Dr. X says.

"And that," I say, "is a delay before the onset of treatment." Dr. X nods.

"So," Jenelle says, "will an additional month or more be detrimental to his condition?"

Dr. X sighs. "You're putting me in an awkward spot with that question. I'll just say this: If it were me, and I had exactly what he has, progressed to this point, I'd want to start treatment as soon as possible."

"So a month is bad?" says Jenelle.

"This can be a fairly aggressive form of cancer," Dr. X responds. "More delay certainly cannot help."

There comes a pause.

"I've got to be honest with you, Dr. X. I don't know what to do. How much radiation are we talking about?"

"About six weeks, every day, Monday through Friday. And two, possibly three chemo treatments, each twenty-one days apart."

"How soon could I start? If I wanted to get treated here, I mean."

"If you want to be treated here, we can sign you up for the next available slot to get set up for radiation. Maybe a few days."

Jenelle and I pepper Dr. X with more questions. She patiently answers. Doctor X has me 75% convinced to stick here with her, so I go ahead and have her schedule a consultation with Dr. The Man regarding radiation treatment. He has an opening for next Tuesday, the eighth of January, only three business days away.

After I get the appointment with Dr. The Man, I hang my head in my hands. I look up. "I'm still not 100% sure, but for now I'm leaning toward you. I'll cancel that appointment if I decide differently."

"Well, why don't you sleep on it? Call me when you *do* decide."

* * *

Kaily and I arrive at our taekwondo school. This will be the first class I've been to since December 12. I really miss this class—it's like popping the bottom out of the Stress Bucket, which looks like Old Faithful right now. Class goes well and I feel great. As exercise goes, the escalator stair machine is a form of torture, while taekwondo is fun and requires skill. No matter how many times I suffer for twenty minutes on the stair machine, or at what level, taekwondo is more rigorous. I'm exhausted – and I am calm for the first time in days.

The Next Morning

I've been warned by Dr. X not to Google my diagnosis or prognosis or anything else related to cancer, but I am an engineer and cannot help myself. To help make the big decision over which treatment facility to use, I enter the search strings "prognosis, BSCC" and "BSCC cancer." In the articles that appear, the words "rare" and "highly aggressive" pop up like Whack-a-Moles. My favorite phrase is "poor survival outcomes." One article says that the five-year survival rate for BSCC is "substantially" lower than that for garden variety Squamous Cell Carcinoma (SCC). The reason given is distant metastases (up to six times higher incidence thereof for BSCC). Finally I stumble upon a study that shows that BSCC patients have death rates no worse than SCC patients. Woo hoo!

But overall, the consensus seems to be that Lumpy the BSCC marauder waits for no man—and he doesn't just dribble out metastases, he catapults them. A month of delays seems out of the question. Google just demolished all the calm I found after taekwondo class.

But a thought occurs: While it seems like delay after delay, the reality is that I have created no delays whatsoever in the local cancer center's schedule. Things are proceeding there as fast as they would be without all the worry, so why worry? I already have an appointment with Dr. The Man.

Relax, I tell myself. If only it were that easy.

Sunday, January 6

Carina, blissfully unaware of my inner turmoil, returns to Rice. She and Kaily see me coming back from the gym, and Kaily goes to taekwondo with me, so they both continue to figure that we have this thing fully under control.

Kaily and I ice skate at the Houston Aerodrome, and for a couple of hours I do not think about cancer at all. I try to knock the rust off of my backward skating abilities, and she laughs because I wipe out—a few times.

"If you're not fallin'," I say, "you're not tryin'!"

"Yeah, right," she says.

While tryin' a massive ice-throwing hockey-style two-skate stop from full speed, I fall on my tailbone, bruising it badly.

Kaily finds this hilarious. "How old are you, again?"

January 7

Dr. X's nurse calls me back after I leave two messages on her answering machine. I tell her that I am now good and ready to start treatment, and for her to please schedule me for chemo ASAP, just in case I want it. But I might cancel it. I mention how we engineers believe in contingency plans. I tell her that I will keep my appointment with Dr. The Man tomorrow regarding radiation treatment, just in case I want that as well. She takes all this down and informs me that one can schedule neither chemo nor radiation on a contingency basis. She wants me to get back to her once I make an actual decision. Some engineer she is.

"Tomorrow," I say. "Maybe."

Kaily and I return for another taekwondo class; it is hugely rigorous, but I survive. I do forty-six pushups in forty-five seconds, with elbows tucked in tightly and good form all the way up and all the way down. This gives me hope and calms me until bedtime, as my subconscious mind connects pushup quantity with cancer vanquishing.

It takes a long time to get to sleep, over an hour, because of the thinking. I lay face up, obsessing about beginning treatment. Jenelle, too, has Googled articles about BSCC, and by now has scared herself into wanting me to start treatment right away. Empathy at last.

The Pole

I have owned lots of cars. I keep a spreadsheet documenting them – make, model, years of ownership, year sold, etc.—because I am an engineer. The tally is up to twenty-four since I started driving in 1980, but usually Jenelle will only let me keep two at any given time (*Women...*).

In our household, cars have names: The Cop Car (an exhighway patrol car); The Pink Lady ('72 Chevy pickup with a 400-horsepower big block, covered in rust and primer faded to pink); The Blue Cloud ('82 Olds 98 Regency). My current daily driver is The Penguin, a white Chevy Trailblazer Super Sport with black interior. It resembles, to Kaily, a penguin. She has a point. The Penguin is fairly new, with less than 30,000 miles on it.

This morning I drive The Penguin to work, where time passes glacially. But I finally log off my Firm D computer for the day. This afternoon is my initial consultation with Dr. The Man, radio oncologist extraordinaire. I cannot wait. I ponder treatment venue decisions, and how I must now drive The Penguin across town through rush-hour traffic for my consultation. I stop in at the men's room prior to leaving the building.

Once when I was in a gym locker room, a man was standing in front of a urinal, one hand on action central, the other holding a cell phone to his ear. As he pissed heartily, he had a romantic conversation with his significant other.

"Oh, yeah, Baby, I can't wait for dinner either." Piss, piss. "What are you going to wear? Mmm, hmmm...oh yeah, I love that skirt. You know how it makes me..." Piss, piss. "Yeah, I'm sure looking forward to *that!*" Piss, piss, trickle, trickle. "Okay, Baby, got to go now. Love you!" Click. Flush.

Observing Urinal Romeo at the gym established my policy of no phone contact while gripping the organ; instead I just let calls roll to phone mail. Enter Lumpy. I'm in mid-stream in Firm D's men's room when the phone rings. I panic and grab the phone with my free hand to check who's calling. It is Ms. Helpful from MDA. Before answering, I finish the piss but do not flush, as I do not want to give away the scene. The silent subtext of my conversation goes like this: "I am not standing before a urinal" and "There is no male organ in my other hand."

"Hello," I say out loud.

"Hello, David," she says, "I have more news."

The urinal, as it turns out, has an automatic sensor with incredible timing. There is a loud flush.

"Uhm," Ms. Helpful murmurs, "should I call back?"

"No, yeah, well, sorry, it's just that I saw it was you and decided to answer."

"I'm not sure how to reply to that."

"Oh, I don't mean that... it's just that I'm anxious for news. Anyhow, I'm finished now."

"Uhm, we'd better talk later."

"No! Oh, sorry, no, I'm good."

I wash my hands, making yet more bathroom racket. She thankfully continues anyway, and I am able to make my escape from the men's room before any more embarrassing noises can erupt.

After reviewing my files, MDA feels that it is not a "head and neck" problem, but an "unknown origin" problem. My case, therefore, will be transferred to the GI (Gastro-Intestinal) department.

"What? Why there?"

"Because," she explains, "they're the ones who deal with unknown origin. Furthermore, they won't touch your case until they receive the actual pathology slides from the lymph node sample. Also, if MD Anderson looks at your slides and you do not come here for treatment, there will be a two hundred and fifty dollar fee per slide, with a $2500 maximum. Do you know how many slides you have?"

"I have no idea," I say, "but you're telling me that I could spend $2500 and have MDA tell me the same thing that I already know?"

"Yes."

"What about the possible skin cancer connection? What does MDA feel about that? Why the GI department?"

"Because," Ms. Helpful says, "theories carry no weight. Only slides matter. Get us those slides and we'll proceed. If you like, we can request your slides for you."

This is all too much and I tell Ms. Helpful to do nothing until I call her back. I need time to think this over.

I ponder the objective and scientific manner in which MDA is going about their business. As an engineer, I find it to be quite logical. As someone who wants to commit premeditated and immediate Lumpy-cide, I find it to be a load of horse shit.

I phone Jenelle (not in the presence of any bathroom fixtures) and relay the developments. It turns out that she has continued to obsess over yet more Internet articles about BSCC. She also feels compelled to tell me what she has read: stories of death, misdiagnosis, misreading of slides, and various details involving the word "hyper-aggressive." She informs me that she is stressed out and in bad mental shape.

"How do you think I feel?" I bark. There is silence in reply. "Sorry," I say. "Look, I have to go, let me call you from the car."

"Okay," she sighs.

I hurry down to the parking lot. The day is rainy, misty, nasty. For the entire walk to The Penguin, I feel conflict raging inside my head. One of my female coworkers, M, talks on the cell phone out where the smokers smoke. I wave on my way past her.

I start The Penguin and begin the mental churning. I'm nearly "in" at MDA, although there will be a huge delay in treatment if I go there. But they're the best! (Maybe.) But it's aggressive cancer. Then again, it could cost $2500 just to get the slides looked at.... Radiation? When do I want it? Now! No, I should wait for MDA...

I take the back way out of the parking lot, the same way I've been leaving since I started to work at Firm D. I begin to round a corner by a tin roof that serves as covered parking for several spots. My mind is moonwalking while juggling chainsaws. I look around and see no cars or pedestrians, then glance down for my cell phone so I can finish my call with Jenelle.

BOOM! The outside mirror to my left explodes. I hear a cruel screech and rending of metal down the length of the car. I have no idea what just happened other than me becoming instantly confused, so I jam on the brakes and come to a stop. Reflexively looking for the mirror, I see it hanging off the door like an eyeball dangling by the optic nerve. I try to open the door, but it fights back with more screeching and rending, so of course I try harder. As it gives way, it occurs to me that I have just wrecked the shit out of my car. I step out for a visual confirmation.

"What the hell did I just hit?" I say aloud to no one.

I look back in the misty rain and there it is: a steel pole, four feet tall, six inches in diameter and filled with concrete. The outside of the pole is the color of rust, now decorated with a stripe of white paint from The Penguin. I have no idea how this pole jumped in my way; I certainly do not recall seeing it before. I check out The Penguin. Its front fender is smashed, front wheel askew, driver's door trashed, mirror still dangling by a cable. I've managed to scrape, bend, or dent each panel from bow to stern, including the rear bumper.

One seldom actually sees a jaw drop open in surprise, but there it is on M's face. She gapes at me from fifty feet away with a mixture of shock and horror, phone held out in her extended left hand, presumably in mid-call. I look at her and back at the car.

Oh, God, my radiation appointment! I look at M again, then back at my car. I don't know what to do. Then I do. I'm driving it the way it is.

"I just wrecked my car!" I yell.   I can practically hear the reply inside M's head, though her mouth remains soundlessly open: *No shit, Captain Obvious!*

"I have to go!" I say. "See you later!" Still, she says nothing.

I pull the handle but the door won't open. I yank harder, putting my weight into it. There's a third chorus of screech-and-rend. I hop into the driver's seat and slam the door closed with more sound effects. The slam violently bounces the mirror, knocking loose a few more bits of glass. I put the poor wounded Penguin in Drive and go. Her steering wheel immediately pulls hard to the left and the driver's front tire begins to squeal as I inch forward. The rain comes down harder.

Oh hell, oh shit... dammit, what have I done? I am in no condition to be driving. Where did that f-ing pole come from? I'll kill myself if I keep driving in this flooded-Bucket state, but I have to get to the cancer center! Remain calm! Wait, I wasn't calm to begin with!

On the spot, I come up with a mantra to keep me focused and to avoid thinking about cancer treatment options. The mantra is a simple question followed by a simple answer, repeated many times in rapid succession: Drivin' the car? *Drivin' the car.* Drivin' the car? *Drivin' the car.*

I pull out into traffic. Drivin' the car? *Drivin' the car.* The mirror slaps the door, the front tire squeals, the steering wheel pulls. I calculate that it is twenty miles from here to Dr. The Man. Squeal, slap, pull. Drivin' the car? *Squeeeal!*

I take the service road because the freeway is out of the question with my car and my mind in this shape. About a third of the way to the cancer center, the smell of burning rubber begins to emerge from The Penguin's vents. Smellin' rubber? *Smellin' rubber.* I decide to slow down or risk blowing the tire out. I am now going thirty miles an hour. Panic comes in waves—am I doing the right thing? Will I even make it to the cancer center? But I have to, because I have to start treatment!

When I'm not busy panicking, I feel a *nouveau* variety of nausea, the kind that comes with the wrecking of one's own Penguin. The mirror slaps and rain comes down. At least my wipers work. Five miles out I think to check my inside rearview mirror. Behind me is a line of cars worthy of a parade. Blockin' traffic? *Blockin' traffic.* There are other lanes on the service road, but it's rainy and people seem cautious, or confused, or perhaps fascinated that The Penguin is managing to roll forward under its own power. They want to see what happens next.

With some freakishly good luck at red lights, timing works out. Pulling into the cancer center parking lot only five minutes late, I bend the car door open and hop out. A small amount of smoke pours from what's left of the tire.

"Sorry, Baby," I say, patting a smashed fender. I hope she won't catch fire, but figure that if she does, the rain will put her out. I run to the building.

Doctor The Man

I skid into the waiting room and sign in, wet and breathless. People stare. TV News blares from the big screen. Not just TV news, but Fox News, i.e. "newsertainment." I am in hell.

Jenelle rises from a couch. "How come you're late?"

I can't even begin to answer. The world's against me; she must be against me. But she probably asked that question because I'm almost always on time, or early. That is, unless I'm singlehandedly wrecking my own car. She reaches up and turns the TV off. She's with me after all, and is also an angel from heaven.

At this point, any last shards of sanity should be gone, but I look around and see a half dozen cancer patients awaiting their turns. Some have hair, and some not, which I surmise from the array of scarves and hats. Their stoicism restores my perspective. The Penguin as well, has brought me to my appointment, ignoring her own pain and suffering to get me here. She's Trigger, Lassie, and one of those smart, TV dolphins. I breathe a few deep ones....

Wow, did I just calm down after all that? Why, yes, I did. Saved by Jenelle and the Penguin, and the strength of other Cancer Club members.

I sign the usual suite of release forms without reading one of 'em. I fill in the prescription drug form: None. Then come the radiation release forms. These I read and pass on to Jenelle as I finish them. There will be side effects, amongst which could be *cancer*. That's right! In the course of treating cancer via radiation, tissue damage may occur, showing up years later in the form of cancer. Also "possible" as in Very Likely: fatigue, loss of appetite, nausea, low red and white-cell counts, sore throat, weight loss, tissue loss, radiation rash, depression, anger, helplessness, scarring of sensitive tissue, difficulty in thinking, short-term memory loss, and hair loss.

Jenelle and I finish reading the list of side effects. "Yadda, yadda, yadda," I say. "Sign my ass up!"

Jenelle is less enthusiastic. She reminds me of her father's "one last radiation treatment," when he came out with swollen lungs and an oxygen tank that he was forced to use until his death. But the listed side effects are the price of my future which, at the moment, I do not feel that I have much of. I sign everything and hand it back in.

I hear a man discussing his insurance with the receptionist. She explains that because the cancer hospital is new, they are still negotiating with the insurance company for coverage.

" So," the man says, "I may not be covered?"

"Oh, you probably will," she answers.

This does not inspire confidence. The man sits back down and I ask him who his insurance company is. He sees my card out and says, "The same as yours."

Jenelle and I are called into the back and led to an exam room. A nurse enters carrying a laptop. She sits and begins asking me questions. I glance over and notice that her software is called "Oncochart." She takes down symptoms, diagnoses, family history, information about who I've seen and what I've done so far for the cancer, and more. This seems quite organized and gives us comfort. The nurse wraps it up and leaves.

After a brief wait a female doctor, perhaps five feet tall, enters. She introduces herself as Dr. Fi, radio oncologist. She sports gray hair, an infallible sign of experience, thus making her my dream doctor. Dr. Fi goes over my Oncochart entries and listens to my story from the beginning. She is patient and quite attentive, interested in my entire cancer monologue.

While I speak, she feels the lymph nodes around my throat, and then feels Lumpy. She checks around my body for other swollen lymph nodes. She says that she agrees with the selection of tests I have thus far endured, and mentions that the only other diagnostic tool she can think of would be a bronchoscopy, similar to the thin, snake-like camera my ENT used to poke around in my sinuses. There is a special version of this snake for the lungs, and it gives a visual confirmation of PET scan results. Dr. Fi listens to my lungs with a stethoscope and says that I may or may not be asked to go through the bronchoscopy, depending on the opinion of Dr. The Man.

He enters.

Dr. The Man looks over the Oncochart and begins to ask questions—no nonsense, just this side of terse. He feels various lymph nodes while he interrogates, then pulls out his stethoscope and listens to my lungs. Dr. Fi mentions that the only test I have not yet undergone is a bronchoscopy. Dr. The Man listens some more and frowns. Before I can take this in the worst way possible, he says, "No. No bronchoscopy indicated."

Dr. Fi looks at me as if to say, *Well, then!* I exchange glances with Jenelle.

Dr. The Man lays me down on the exam table and examines my testicles. I ponder a remark like, "Not even so much as a kiss first?" but resist the urge. I don't want to offend a person in such a position of power over my life, nor do I want him to take me up on it. He pronounces my testicles free of Lumpy relatives, which I find to be a far greater relief than I had anticipated.

He and Dr. Fi confer, and then decide that they concur with each other and with Dr. X. The treatment regimen stands as written: multitudinous zaps of radiation interspersed with squirts of caustic chemicals. Dr. The Man blows out of the room, leaving a wake of authoritative confidence and happy testes.

Dr. Fi stays behind with Jenelle and me. "Dr. Fi," I say, "it sounds like we're all set. When can we start?"

"We shall begin the planning right away," she replies.

I look at Jenelle and back at Dr. Fi. "Rock and roll!" I exclaim.

"Excuse me?" Dr. Fi says.

"Oh, I mean, let us commence. Do proceed."

Dr. Fi explains that she will coordinate the details of the radiation treatment, while Dr. X will remain as the overall coordinator, including chemo arrangements.

Dr. Fi takes her pen and points toward Lumpy's lair.

"You will receive a dose of radiation concentrated upon the cancer in your left axilla." She draws an ever widening circle in the air with her pen. "The radiation is quite concentrated in a small area, and will become rapidly weaker as the distance extends away." Poking at my neck, she adds, "The affected region will end at your neck, but will not extend into your lungs."

She walks behind me and draws a circle with her finger around my left shoulder. Jenelle watches beside her. "Around here, the treatment will extend from the shoulder down toward your scapula, and might affect muscles as far away as here." Now Dr. Fi pokes me in the left lat muscle, which tickles, making me giggle like the Pillsbury Dough Boy.

I am happy to hear of this radius of destruction around Lumpy, but become concerned about my athletic future. "Will it...will the radiation destroy this shoulder joint?"

"Oh, no, no," she says. "The radiation will destroy the cancer, but will only damage the muscle and connective tissue. These will recover and you should regain much if not all of the use of your shoulder."

This I find nearly as welcome as the news about the testicles. I'm about to ask if I can keep exercising when she adds,   "There will, however, be side effects. First off, you cannot use that shoulder during the term of radiation treatment, nor for a month afterward. Oh, I mean you can use it, but you cannot expose it to rigorous exercise, as the radiation causes inflammation and possible weakness. You could damage that shoulder with overuse. Also, there will be a rash, like sunburn, on the affected area."

I ask her about the release form and its other listed side effects. She nods her head.

"Yes, all of that is possible. I think in your case, you will feel a bit dizzy at times, and possibly quite tired."

Jenelle and I exchange looks yet again. I expect her to say something like, "Don't worry, David is usually dizzy," but she does not.

Dr. Fi further explains that there will be an X-ray and a special CT scan required. "The physicists will take this data and formulate a series of trajectories, so that the radiation head of the machine can aim at the cancer from various angles."

"Physicists?" Jenelle says.

"Yes, physicists." Dr. Fi turns back toward me. "You will remain fixed, and the head of the radiation machine will traverse around you. At each stop of the head, the angle must be precisely calculated so that the concentrated portion of the beam is aimed directly at the cancer. The treatment regimen will be six weeks, five days per week. Each visit will take approximately forty-five minutes, and the actual radiation itself will last around twenty minutes, give or take."

According to Doc Fi, this type of radiation therapy is called IMRT (Intensity Modulated Radiation Therapy). As the head of the radiation machine is stationed at various places relative to my body, the intensity and pattern of the radiation is modulated. This allows a precise, high-strength dose to be focused on the tumor, while minimally damaging non-cancerous tissue.

"When's the first zap?" I ask, forgetting in the excitement of the moment about this all being a contingency.

"We will schedule your CT scan and X-ray right away," she says. "Possibly this afternoon if we can fit you in." She disappears to see if she can work me into the CT scan queue. The X-ray is a sure thing, as they have their own machine here in the radio-oncology department.

Dr. Fi comes back with the head radio-oncology nurse, Nurse Wonder Woman. Nurse WW is five-foot four-inches of pure Texan, complete with tenacious grit, go-get-'em energy, and full-blown accent. "Don't y'all worry, we'll git 'ya fixed up!"

Dr. Fi goes off to make arrangements from her end, and Nurse WW takes us with her. We go straight to the X-ray machine, which is supposed to mimic the radiation machine. In front of the machine is a stainless slab of a table. I am told to lie down upon the slab.

Nurse WW looks over my information. Dr. Fi returns and explains to her where the cancer is and what the radiation plan will be. I am on my back, and they scoot me here and there on the table, eventually settling on a position that, if performed standing up, could best be described as Underwear Model. I have my legs straight out, my right hand where my belt buckle would be if I weren't wearing a hospital gown, and my left hand on my left hip. They decide that a pillow is needed, and put one beneath my knees. Nurse WW and Dr. Fi enter the control room and shoot an X-ray.

Nurse WW returns, tells me to sit up and remove the gown. She lays me back into position and says, "I see you got no tattoos."

"That's right," I say.

"Well," she says, "you're fixin' to have some now!"

She pulls out a tattoo machine and tells me to hold still. Red laser beams from above mark spots on my body—one on my shoulder, one in the middle of my chest, and one by my left nipple. She sees something she does not like and puts the tattoo machine down. She and Dr. Fi go back into the control room.

"Don't you move!" comes over a speaker.

"Okay," I reply, wondering if she can hear me.

After another X-ray, Nurse WW and Dr. Fi reenter the room.

Nurse WW picks up the tattoo machine and hovers over my chest.

"Are those tattoos henna?" Jenelle says.

"No, ma'am. They're the real McCoy." Nurse WW then proceeds to give me three tattoos, each a black dot the size a well-inked ballpoint pen might leave.

"Those aren't very impressive," I say. "Can you draw a big snake, maybe holding a machine gun?"

"What kinda' snake you want?" she grins, and leans over again.

"He was joking," Jenelle says. "I think."

Nurse WW puts the tattoo gear away and disappears around the corner. She reappears with a flat piece of white plastic mesh in a three-sided frame, roughly the shape of a horse shoe (for a big freaking Clydesdale). Drops of water fall from the mesh.

"What are you going to do with that?" I ask.

"Pull it down over your face," she says.

I think that she is joking and laugh. "Ha, ha, no, really."

"Hold still and look straight up," she instructs. I do so and she pulls the hot wet mesh down over my face. It forms a net over my entire head. She attaches the frame to the stainless slab with some small bolts. She molds the wet mesh around my nose, and presses it to the contours of my face.

"Comfortable?" she says.

"Huh?" I ask. I can't remember the last time I was actually comfortable.

"Is your *face* comfortable?"

The mesh makes it difficult to speak. "I gueff," I respond, even though I'm not comfortable at all.

"Good!" she says, "'Cause that mesh is fixin' to harden. You'll be wearin' this mask durin' every radiation treatment. Don't move."

I don't move, and the mask begins to harden. "Ith kinda tight in here," I say, through unmoving jaws.

"You'll get used to it," Nurse WW informs me.

Dr. Fi comes into my line of sight and tells me that she was able to get me into the CT-scan machine tomorrow, Wednesday, January 9. That will be the last procedure prior to turning my information over to the physicists for aiming the radiation machine.

The mask has hardened, and Nurse WW finally unbolts me from the stainless slab. "Alrighty, see y'all tomorrow!" I thank her for unbolting my face and move my jaw a few times. The mask, constrictive as it was, now seems like only the slightest annoyance. Finally I feel like treatment is coming, and I am ecstatic. Jenelle is happy. Dr. Fi is happy too, and can sense my excitement.

"Rock and roll?" Dr. Fi says.

"Rock and roll!" I confirm.

* * *

Jenelle follows me to the auto body shop, which is fortunately only a couple of miles from the cancer center. I pull up—the tire is smoking again—and am greeted by the owner.

"Dude!" he yells, looking at The Penguin. "What the hell did you do?" I explain about the pole. "Oh, that sucks!"

"Yeah, crappy luck."

"Not your luck, man, your car! This thing is practically brand new!" He takes it all in then looks up at me. "Dude," he says, staring at my face. "What the hell did you do?"

"What do you mean? I just told you. I hit a pole."

"No, dude, I mean your face!"

"What?"

I walk over to the mirror, but it's dangling to the side and has no glass left in it, so I walk to the other side and look in that mirror. My face, and especially my forehead, is covered in an evenly spaced diamond pattern of red indentations. "It's a long story," I sigh. I just don't have the energy to explain.

We go over the damage. He says he'll need body parts, lots of body parts. Basically, the entire driver's side will be replaced or repaired, and all of it repainted; it may not require a new wheel, but will definitely require some suspension and alignment work and a tire. Needs a new mirror, of course, and maybe some things he cannot yet determine. While he talks, I take a picture of The Penguin with my cell phone. I tell him to call me when he figures out how long the repair will take.

Jenelle drives me home. We have mixed emotions. She is happy that treatment might begin soon, but I cannot tell if she is fully on board with the local treatment center or not. I decide not to ask, just in case her answer does not match my own desire. I finally have Lumpy in my sights, targeted for destruction.

Does that mean I've formally decided on the treatment venue? Not quite.

5 TREATMENT BEGINS

The next day, January 9, I make a cup of coffee and step into my office with my journal:

For the rest of the day I suffered manic depression. On moment I'd be up (as the doctors had concurred) and the next down (treatment STILL won't begin until next Monday with chemo possibly by Tuesday). Yet another week will pass. It was like when Kaily went to the orthodontist expecting her braces to be removed, only to find out that she'd have to get bottom braces added, and keep the whole conglomeration for another year. Note that Sunday will mark one month since my lymph-node operation... Lance was treated within only days. Me? One month. Don't get cancer over Christmas... I cannot overstate my impatience and depression over the delays.

I go to Firm D, and mention to Armchair that I hit a pole in the parking lot. "It was the freakiest thing," I say. "I mean, I honestly can't remember that pole being there."

"That's because it wasn't," Armchair says. "They just installed that thing over the weekend. It's brand new."

Minutes later I stand in the parking lot, staring at the pole. It is now covered in bright yellow safety tape, and has a cone in front of it. *Interesting timing*, I think. None of the decorations were there when I hit it. Later I send an email to the office manager asking how to get hold of the owners of the building, as Firm D is only a renter. I receive an email address, and send a message to the building owners explaining my situation. They don't bother to email back, ever. Normally this sort of thing would send me through the roof and I would pursue Justice at all costs, but I cannot work up any energy to fight it. I have car insurance, and being more worried about Death than Justice, I just chalk it up to one more shitty thing about getting cancer.

I am now in my office at home. Today I am rid of the mania, sinking firmly into depression. It is an ebb tide of optimism. Out of dumb habit I open my email. There's a new one from an aunt in Ohio telling me how wonderful the news is about my PET scan results, and how happy we must all be. Two percent of my brain shares the sentiment. The rest just wants to kill Lumpy right now, somehow, or sleep for five days straight.

As I close the email from my aunt, the phone rings. It is Ma. Instead of "Hello" or, "How are you feeling today, good son?" she opens with "You *have* to get a second opinion! You *need* to go to MD Anderson!"   While she continues the monologue, I can't help remembering the title of Rodney Dangerfield's autobiography: *It Ain't Easy Being Me.*

Normally Ma and I can duke it out for quite a few rounds, but I am too sapped to fight. Before hanging up, she informs me that she has explained my entire case to our good family friend, and my ex-pediatrician, Doc Kid.

"Doc Kid says you're making a mistake, too! He wants you to call him, right away!"

She gives me his number. I can only imagine Ma's version of my medical condition: brain tumors on the march, seeping wounds, missing limbs.... I lay on the floor working up the strength to call Doc Kid. My mood swings ever so slightly back toward okay, and I climb to my desk to make the call.

"Hello, David?" he says. "Your mother told me all about the quacks down at your local cancer center and how they have a bizarre unique mystery diagnosis that no one's ever heard of. It sounds like they don't know what they're doing. You have to get a second opinion. You have to go to MD Anderson!"

Et tu, Doc Kid?

Doc Kid and I have a long conversation. I consult my notes and give him all the details. By the end he has calmed down, tentatively agreeing that I might be pursuing a good course of action on my own. He is buddies with an oncologist, and will ply the man for information and advice. He'll call me back. I tell him thanks, because I am awfully stressed out, and more information will certainly be helpful. I hang up and put my head in my hands. I try to decide whether to be happy or depressed. The choice is too difficult.

"Daddy?" It is Kaily. She has been listening just outside the door. She steps in. "Daddy, I heard you say that you're stressed out." I look up and nod. She looks concerned momentarily, but then gets the proverbial twinkle in her eye. "I know what to do," she says.

Before I can say something like, "Not now, Kaily! I want to keep stressing out alone!" she exclaims, "Chocolate and Hawaiian music!"

This is a sufficiently oddball suggestion that it throws me off my game; now I'm curious. She hops out of the room and walks right back in carrying a small tray laden with various types of chocolate from the girls' emergency reserve stash. She has me fire up the Internet radio, and we tune in some tranquil Hawaiian music. I listen and think of trade winds and chocolate melting in the hot sun. Blue skies and blue water, breaking waves...It's working! Kaily should hang up her shingle as a Stress Reduction Specialist. She'd make a million.

Pre-Radiation CT Scan

After the Hawaiian Cocoa therapy, the world seems a better place. I feel a bit of strength return and suddenly remember that it's time for my pre-radiation CT scan.

I report, as instructed, to the same office where I underwent my PET scan. The CT scan machine in here is special, in that it has a slab, which mimics the one I'll be attached to during radiation.

The old Hispanic woman at the receptionist's desk recognizes me; I am becoming a regular customer. "Hello, Mr. Hewitt!" She hands me a stack of paperwork. I sign each form without reading it.

Nurse WW blasts through the doors to the waiting room. She pushes a cart with various items on it, one of which I recognize: My new mesh face mask.

"Hey, y'all!" she says. "Ready to get this thing going?"

I look at the mask and it looks dumbly back at me. "What do you think?" I say to the mask. "Shall we?" It does not answer.

* * *

I remove my shirt and sit on the stainless slab in front of the CT machine. Ms. Pet Scan is working blood duty again.

"Hi," I say.

"Hi," she replies in a businesslike manner while preparing her needle kit. She seems to not recognize me; must have been a long day in the injection line. I hold out my arm. "Oh!" she squeals, eyes locked onto a blood vessel. "You're my pipeline vein man!"

I have to admit that I'm becoming quite fond of all the attention from the female phlebotomist contingent. This must be how the head stud feels at the thoroughbred farm. Ms. Pet Scan hooks up the iodine IV.

Testicles, make ready! I think. *You dudes have been getting a lot attention lately.*

Nurse WW bolts me down via mesh face mask to the slab. She places a pillow under my knees and has me assume the Recumbent Male Underwear Model pose. The CT machine has no laser guidance lights like those on the imitation radiation machine, so Nurse WW has to run me in and out—I count five trips—tweaking my position each time. Finally I am in the proper position and the scan begins. The machine spools up, the red lights rotate about me, the gurney moves in and out, and I stare at the Phillips-head screws. The mask is noticeably harder than the night before when she fit me with it. I feel a wave of claustrophobia; I am trapped. This mask would make a great centerpiece for a bad horror story:

Our irradiated hero flails at the cruel bolts, but his arms, lustily veined as they are, cannot reach them—the bolts mock him, holding his head fast in a mask of grim claustrophobic torture. Nurse WW has been replaced by her evil twin, Nurse Evil, who is on a psychotic high after chugging a radioactive cocktail of PET scan goo, berry delicious contrast, and Cisplatin. She approaches him with a mischievous grin and an idling chain saw...

The mesh digs into my Adam's apple. The chainsaw-toting nurse could have her way with me and I could hardly make a peep. But thankfully the CT scan is quite brief. Instead of a full-body scan, it is concentrated only on Lumpy, the bastard!

Nurse WW comes to unbolt my face. "Comfy in there?" she inquires.

My lower jaw is even more constrained than before, so I talk like a ventriloquist. "The mesh if digging into my froat," I mumble.

"Oh, that's pretty common when these masks harden up. We can cut it a little if you want."

"Yeah, how about you go ahead and do dat?" I panic, hoping that my words did not come out too angrily, as she has not yet unbolted my face. "Prease," I add. Nurse WW unbolts me, which her evil twin would never do.

I sit up, feeling the indentations in my forehead. "So," I venture, "when can I start radiation?"

Nurse WW looks at the CT machine while she does some calculations in her head. "Most likely, due to the amount of work involved, we can't get you in until Monday."

"Monday?"

"Yep. The physicists have to run their calculations and then program the setup. It can take a while, depending on where you are in line."

I leave the cancer center feeling like a soft-serve ice-cream cone with two flavors, happy and disappointed. I want to start treatment so badly it feels almost like a physical ache, like junior-high love. I imagine Lumpy, the most vile, verminous growth imaginable, residing contentedly in my left axilla, growing and reproducing so that he and his satanic offspring can kill me by the summer solstice. I want that son of a bitch the hell out.

I arrive home and my cell phone rings. It is Ms. Helpful at MD

Anderson. She has transferred my case to GI and needs my insurance card again. It might be possible, she says, for my slide-reading fees to be covered by insurance.

"Also, congratulations," she says, "as you've been accepted as a patient."

"Good freaking timing," I say.

"Excuse me?" she answers. "You haven't begun treatment elsewhere, have you? Because if you have, we have to decline you as a patient."

"I haven't actually begun," I say, "but all the preparations have been made for radiation treatment, and chemo could start next week."

"We have to know then: What's your decision? Here, or there?"

As anxious as I am to begin treatment, the timing of this MDA phone call has me spooked. I have a flash debate in my head:

Ethics aside, the radiation prep work at the local cancer center is still a contingency; it's just an ace in the hole.

But I'm ready for treatment now! Switching would cause delays!

This is MDA we're talking about. Seriously, you could still change your mind right now, right this instant.

Yeah, and there would be some pissed of medical professionals and some heinous bills...for nothing.

What are a few bills? This is a life-or-death decision!

Or is it?

What are you going to do?

What the hell should I do?

Talkin' on the phone?

Talkin' on the phone.

"Let me call you back," I say to Ms. Helpful.

"Okay, but don't wait too long."

I see that my cell phone has new a message on it. It's from my brother in-law: "What's this about you being treated locally? You're right up the road from the best of the best, why don't you use them? We need to talk, bro!"

I know he means well—don't they all? But in my current mood, his tone doesn't help. Fortunately it is only a message and we did not speak live, for the call pisses me off. I have the urge to say, "Yeah, they did a bang-up job on your old man, didn't they? Zero for one, by my scorecard, *bro!*"

Bitterness, anyone? But I resist the urge to call back with that message, instead phoning Jenelle about the incident. She has received a similar message: "What's going on? What are you doing? You need to call here and talk!" We agree that her brother means well, and decide to let it go at that.

I tell Jenelle that I am feeling a lot of pressure about the decision. She listens and is quiet a moment. "I won't pressure you," she says. "The decision is up to you."

We hang up and I ponder this. I decide to take Jenelle up on her offer and make the decision myself. I will not try to please everybody else, or perhaps *anybody* else. This is an epiphany; I feel a nearly physical sensation of weight coming off. I will sleep on it and decide tomorrow.

I attend my last taekwondo class for the foreseeable future. My stomach hurts as I drive up—must be the stress of it all, hope it's not stomach cancer. We begin conditioning and I try hard, completing all of the drills. I find myself a bit more winded than usual.

Then we perform a multitude of kicking drills, which turn out to be a lot of fun; I think nothing about cancer for the rest of the hour. The stomachache fades away but my left hip still hurts, probably leftover inflammation from my wipeout at the ice rink. I bid the school owner, Master Steel Curtain, goodbye for now; he bows and wishes me luck.

We go to bed, and Jenelle falls asleep immediately. I cannot sleep; there are too many voices speaking in my head, so I decide to try the Serenity Prayer. I wait a few seconds for results. Nothing. I think that perhaps once isn't enough; perhaps a dozen times will do. I launch into it, and soon lose count. At first nothing happens, but I keep going anyway. Out of nowhere, maybe ten times into the prayer, calmness descends and I have a moment of clarity. I decide to let it go—all of it—my worry, my decision, other people's opinions, my future. It is all out of my hands; I am not the one driving the bus. I feel better than I've felt in days and fall into a deep sleep lasting until my alarm goes off the next morning.

January 10

Some of the serenity of the previous night lingers, and I have a mellow drive to the office. I feel less concerned than the day before, and am able to work.

I stand before the urinal at Firm D to do my business. My cell phone rings. One might think that my prior experience and new-found serenity would induce me to let the call go. Instead I'm suddenly on a razor's edge and think, *What if it's cancer news?* I pull the phone out of my pocket with my free hand and see that it's the cancer center.

"David?"

I do not recognize the voice. "Yes?"

"Nurse Wonder Woman, here. I've got good news for y'all: it's on like a pot o'neck bones!"

"Uhm, excuse me?"

"Your radiation! It's been moved forward!"

"Really? To when?"

"Today!" she says. "Five o'clock!"

This is good news. I manage to finish the phone call without flushing. The worm has turned, so to speak.

So I get to begin radiation three days early. I am ecstatic—what a break! I will show up at 5:00 and the killing of Lumpy will commence. Decision made, as far as I am concerned. I will begin treatment today and will not go to MDA, the rest of the world be damned. I phone Ms. Helpful at MDA and tell her of my decision. She is not upset or judgmental in any way. "We can't touch you now, though," she says. "However, if in the future you get recurrence, or a different cancer crops up, you can always re-apply."

That makes me feel all warm and happy inside, almost like an iodine bath for the boys. "Wow, thanks!" I say.

"Good luck," she responds.

* * *

I'm home early and call Jenelle to tell her the news. I pick up the phone but do not hear a dial tone. I look at the phone a moment and then just for the hell of it, decide to speak. "Hello?"

"Hello, David?"

It's Dr. X's nurse—I've accidentally picked up the phone before it could even ring. She tells me that my "Chemo-teach" is scheduled for tomorrow. Chemo-teach is Chemo 101, a class taught to newbies like me by the nurse who will administer my treatment. This day just gets better and better. I pull out my journal and jot down the following entry: *Halle-F'ing-lu-jah!*

I eat a snack and a thought occurs to me: the Serenity Prayer works. I make another journal entry:

So by letting go and not worrying about it, it happened on its own—the onset of treatment.

Radiation

Five o'clock rolls around; I hop in Little Blue and put the top down. The weather is perfect—cool and clear. I drive to the cancer center down some back roads. Traffic is light and it's the most pleasant drive I've had in recent memory, maybe ever.

Radiation Row is a line of parking spots for glow-in-the-dark patients of the cancer center. The rest of the lot is full, but there is a single spot open on Radiation Row. Nurse Wonder Woman scored me the special parking pass during my previous visit. The pass is yellow, but it doesn't say "Livestrong." In essence it says, *This poor son of a bitch has to suffer through radiation because he has cancer, so give him some slack and at least let him park close to the door. Odds are he's really old.* Oh, but I'm young and virile and don't really need special parking. Still, I'm a club member now, so I pull into my spot. Membership has its privileges.

I enter the radiation waiting room and meet Dee, the new receptionist. Dee is a gentle woman, slightly graying, warm. Dee has me fill out the same paperwork as always. She says that I may take a seat in the lounge area until I finish working through the pile.

"Not necessary," I say. I blast through the stack in seconds flat.

"Aren't you even going to read it?" she says.

"Again, not necessary. O-P-P, you know."

At first, I am the only one in the waiting room. But then the glass doors from the outside world slowly open and a hunched-over, old woman shuffles in. She is bald and makes no bones about it—no hat, no wig, *nada*. Her smooth pate says *I have cancer, by God, so there!* She finds a seat far from me and stares at her sturdy shoes.

The furniture is comfy and homey—a few couches and stuffed arm chairs, all in warm hues. The place is expensively decorated, but not ostentatiously so. A large-screen TV hangs in the corner, blaring CNN. Nobody watches. I look around at the magazine selection: there is a cancer magazine, a cancer magazine of a different name, and the same cancer magazine from last fall. I pick one up and begin to thumb through the cheery articles: *Post-Amputation Do's and Don'ts, Yoga Positions for Low Cell Counts, Advances in Reconstructive Lower GI Surgery, Dealing with Feeling: Your Spouse's Demise, Fun Blender Recipes for Asparagus.* It's a whole new world!

Nurse WW comes in, full of energy and competence. "How're you?"

"Doin' well, thanks."

"Let's get after it!" She guides me to the door of the men's changing room. "Just take your shirt off, darlin', and leave them pants on. There's a clean gown folded up in each cubby—just pick one and put 'er on. Come on out the back door and there's a special little waiting room for you. After treatment, just wad that gown up and put it in the bin by the door."

I walk through the door to find a narrow locker room with four curtained cubicles. I hang my shirt on a hook and put on the gown. Otherwise I am fully dressed, including belt with metal buckle, shoes, and wedding ring. My pockets are full of wallet, car keys, and cell phone. I ponder how radioactive all this will become, remembering that I had to remove it all for my PET and CT scans.

I exit another door and find a tiny waiting room with two seats separated by a narrow table. There is a TV spewing a shrill cable-news assault from the opposite wall. I find the remote on the narrow table and turn it off. I pick up yet another cancer magazine and have just begun to read *Sex, Chemo, and You,* when Nurse WW comes to collect me.

She leads me down a curved linoleum corridor, eventually turning through a wide opening in the wall. "Hold on," she says, and runs back out for something.

I am left alone in an alcove, standing before a wall of shelves. The shelves are filled with mesh face masks, which makes me think of skulls in an Italian catacomb. *How many of us will die?* I get a chill and then regain composure. *All of us. We just don't know when.* These masks represent a lot of cancer patients, especially for such a new, relatively small cancer facility. Nurse WW comes back in carrying nothing and leads me around the corner.

There sits The Beast.

The Beast

My strongest first impression? Is it the size of the hulking mammoth or the foreboding, battleship-gray paint job? The massive radiation head, or the stainless slab upon which I will lay? None of the above. All I want to know is: Why is the hood open on that thing, and what are those people fixing in there?

Two women are working on The Beast, one on a ladder. I hear a medium-sized *bang* such as one might make by striking a piece of sheet metal with a hammer. I do not fancy the idea of anyone banging on this machine, especially just before they strap me down by the face and zap me with it. I try to resist the urge, but cannot; my mouth moves before I can stop it. "And this is supposed to inspire me with confidence?" My sardonic inquiry comes out a bit too loudly; the women working on The Beast stop what they are doing and stare at me, unamused.

When they've completed their work, the hood is closed and they leave the room. What if I pissed them off? What if they have gone off laughing and conspiring: *We'll show that smartass a thing or two—just make sure we remember to swap those wires back before the next patient!*

"Well," says Nurse WW, "Looks like we're ready! Saddle up!"

I walk over to the stainless slab. The lair of The Beast is a nondescript hospital arena with a linoleum floor beneath a ceiling of white acoustical tiles interspersed with fluorescent lights. Muted sounds of cooling fans fill the room. The Beast is huge and industrial, ready to drive off under its own power to find and destroy the puny humans who have rebelled against the Terminator society.

Suddenly the women who had been working under the hood of The Beast reappear. It turns out they are nurses, and they disarm my previous anxiety with warm smiles and friendly introductions. They are calm and reassuring—qualities I value in the last humans I'll see prior to being radioactively molested by a large machine. They instruct me to remove my gown and climb aboard.

The head of The Beast is several feet above and behind me. I lie down and look up. There is a narrow cross, perhaps eight inches to the side, cut from a ceiling tile directly overhead. Laser light falls through the opening and upon me from deep inside the ceiling somewhere. There is a red laser cross slicing me vertically and horizontally across the chest.

Nurse One helps Nurse WW maneuver me into underwear-model position, while Nurse Two bolts my head to the slab. There are no pads on the slab. Nurse WW has eased the harshness ever so slightly by placing a white sheet over the metal. On either side of the slab are stainless steel rods as big around as my thumb, which act as grab handles, ostensibly for hanging onto during panic attacks or any bucking-bronco motions by The Beast. My knees are placed upon a pillow, my face is fixed beneath the mesh, and my left arm is bent with my left thumb tucked into the waistband of my jeans. My left elbow hangs out over the slab—the edge is hard perpendicular steel, and it's quite uncomfortable. My right arm is extended straight toward my hip, the hand grasping a stainless grab bar. I am to hold this position for twenty-odd minutes.

The stainless slab is powered up and elevated. I try to look around but cannot move my head or face, only my eyes. I cannot see my own body. The nurses use the crossing lasers and my tattoos as guides in making adjustments to my position. Nurse One loosens the bolts holding the mask and scoots my head over a half inch. She cranks the bolts back down. Nurse WW scoots my hips over slightly in the opposite direction.

Nurse Two appears above me. "Comfortable?" she says.

"Arrou funkn kidn me?"

She smiles warmly, then disappears from my field of vision. When all is silent I assume that the nurses have left the room for some distant control center—because there's no way they want to be in the same room with all that radiation! That would be crazy!

"We're fixin' to get started," says a voice from a speaker. "I'm about to run the program."

The slab jerks fore and aft slightly, and my elevation shifts slightly. Then nothing else happens.

Nurse One finally appears. "They're not lining up," she says loudly to no one in particular.

"What coordinates are on the sheet?" says the speaker.

Nurse One reads out coordinates. "That's what the console reads," says the speaker.

"Well, they're not lining up."

"Whaf not rhining up?" I mumble.

Nurse One comes into my field of vision and smiles warmly. "Oh, it's all right, Mr. Baskett. The first runs of the program occasionally require a bit of de-bugging."

"A bit uff devugging?" I mumble with alarm.

Nurse WW enters my field of vision. "Relax, y'all, I think someone done transcribed a number wrong. But don't you worry, we have a procedure for finding true zero. This thing'll be dead nuts once I'm through with 'er!"

I do not like hearing the phrase "dead nuts" when I am about to be irradiated. "Now you just sit tight," she says. "We have to take an X-ray."

"I ain goinn any-rare!"

All people not bolted down leave the room. The head of The Beast comes to life, articulating slowly forward and downward, while rotating slightly. The movement is disconcertingly similar to that of a live, intelligent creature. The head maneuvers directly over me, into my line of sight. The underside of the head is flat, about two and a half feet in diameter with a glass lens in the middle, like a large probing eye from an alien spacecraft. The lens is about nine inches across, surrounded by a stainless steel ring held on by eight chromed Phillips head screws (the screw of choice for cancer treatment).

The X-ray is completed, and Nurse WW figures out true zero, then re-enters the coordinates. I remain alone under The Beast. The stainless slab begins to jerk this way and that, and also rises slightly higher in one-centimeter increments. I look into the lens and it stares back at me. I see darkness. I think of a scene from *Jaws* when Quint tells of his ship being sunk in the war:

Sometimes that shark he looks right into ya. Right into your eyes. And, you know, the thing about a shark... he's got lifeless eyes. Black eyes. Like a doll's eyes. When he comes at ya, doesn't seem to be living... until he bites ya, and those black eyes roll over white and then... ah, then you hear that terrible high-pitched screamin'.

There is a brief pause, and through the mesh of my mask I see movement inside the lens. Just on the other side of the glass, two sets of thin, charcoal-colored rectangular bars appear—one set from the far left and one from the far right. They creep slowly toward each other with muted robotic electric motor noises. Each bar is perhaps a tenth of an inch across, a quarter-inch deep, and several inches long. The bars form tightly lined-up rows and look like two dark wooden fences coming together in the middle of the lens. Before the rows collide, some individual bars stop in place; the rest keep coming until they touch. The end result is a jagged crescent moon shape—it's gone from shark to a cat-like pupil, only a bit crooked and jagged, with the bars forming the iris. As Dr. Fi has explained it to me, The Beast would spew forth a wide blast of radiation if not checked; the bars block that which is not needed. The gap left between bars focuses a more precise amount of radiation upon Lumpy, the bastard.

That's all well and good, but I still jump when The Beast's head comes alive again. There are more robotic electric motor sounds as the head traverses around in an arc, rotating about the centerline of my body. It pauses beneath my left shoulder, angled upward (as best as I can see out of the corner of my eye).

I hear a buzz, commensurate with my expectations of how a

radiation machine should sound: like a microwave oven cooking my shoulder. I count. The buzz lasts twenty steamboats (AKA Mississippis, or "seconds" to those not from Ohio).

I look straight up where the head used to be, and in place of the normal acoustical ceiling tiles is a floral scene: wild flowers on a grassy hillside with blue skies and fluffy clouds. It is a photograph printed on plastic panels with light coming through from the other side. The scene is peaceful and serene, and I am suddenly struck with the strange sensation that this horrible room is actually a holy place.

I feel people, or their souls perhaps, all the ones who have lain here hoping, praying, dying or being cured; all wondering. Countless people must have passed through here, strapped to this beast. I have been to a couple places with this same chilling quality of holiness: a shrine outside Santa Fe, and Bergen Belsen in Germany. I've never sat in an electric chair, but I imagine that it's the same kind of cold hardware, retaining ghostly echoes of the souls who have passed—both the guilty and the wrongly accused, all damaged in one way or another. We are all damaged, all guilty of various transgressions against our fellow man. So what am I guilty of? What have I done to deserve this penalty? Maybe plenty, but I settle upon the idea that I'm just unlucky.

There is a pause, a jarring moment of silence, then the head rotates around to the next station, this time to my left, and slightly higher than my shoulder, angled toward the center of my body. I do not like this angle; it looks like The Beast will cook my insides like a cabbage. They must have made a mistake in programming! The mask suddenly feels tighter. I cannot move my head; I am trapped.

I try to calm down. *Stay calm*, I tell myself. Gettin' irradiated? *Gettin' irradiated*. Not the most calming mantra. I can easily imagine a patient losing it, giving in to panic and claustrophobia. I breathe more deeply, but then ease up because I don't want to move in any way that might misdirect the focus of the radiation toward a vital organ. My heart, for example. I say the Serenity Prayer, then say it again. Five more times.

The head rotates slightly about yet another axis. I hear muted electronic motors and see the iris shift slightly. Buzzzz (fifteen steamboats). This continues for a while—the head and neck rotating from behind me, the head itself spinning on its neck, Linda-Blair-like, and the iris shifting each time. Some zaps last fifteen seconds, some thirty, the rest somewhere in between. During and between station changes, time slows down, even seems to stop. It will never end; I have not even finished a single treatment and I have twenty-nine more. How can I find the strength to endure this?

I try to feel the radiation during the pulses. What do I feel? The slab digging into my left elbow, the fatigue of gripping the bar on the right, the tension of trying not to move. I feel my left arm falling asleep, and a slight tingling around Lumpy. Or do I? Can't be sure. Suddenly I realize that the scans and tests have failed to find the tumors in my abdominal cavity. No, there aren't any. *Yes, there are.* Buzzzzz (seventeen steamboats).

It isn't painful, this treatment—not physically. But it *is* psychological torture, by turns calming and excruciating. When I focus on the peculiar holiness of the place and try to put myself in a meditative state, my breathing returns to normal. I fall asleep, perhaps for five or ten seconds, then awaken to more robotic noises, more buzzes.

The head rotates abruptly, ending directly above me; the pupil of The Beast dilates and becomes dead again. The stainless slab lowers. I hear the voices of Nurses WW, One, and Two as they enter the room. Nurse WW starts to unbolt my head and leans into my field of vision. "That wasn't so bad, now was it?"

Lost and Mellow

I find Dr. Fi before changing out of my hospital gown. I tell her that the head of The Beast is angled incorrectly, and is going to cook my internal organs like cabbage. She assures me that it is angled correctly and will not cook me like cabbage. She takes me to the control room, filled with computer monitors and TV monitors showing the lair of The Beast and various other electronic doo-dads. A microphone sits on the desk, making it look like a DJ might sit there. K-HELL: all cancer, all the time!

Dr. Fi shows me a stack of papers containing the programming for The Beast—my programming. She shows me CT scan diagrams of my shoulder, Lumpy included, with "isorads" superimposed in various colors. Isorads form a contour map of how much radiation I am receiving. A red contour directly surrounds Lumpy, indicating a full-strength dose. The colors then taper rapidly off (purple, blue, green, yellow, plaid) as the distance from Lumpy increases. She shows me that "hardly any" radiation will make it to my heart.

"And only thirty percent of that which will kill cancer will make it to a portion of your left lung and your throat."

"Hmm...only thirty percent? Will that damage anything?"

"Oh, nothing permanent," she says.

Normally this would be cause for panic, but my desire to kill Lumpy is so great that I consider a 30% lethal dose of radiation to some of my vital parts to be an excellent tradeoff.

I change back into my shirt and chuck the hospital gown into the hamper. I have worn a tee shirt this day to show off my guns and prove how vital, healthy, athletic and not-going-to-die I am. I can't tell if anyone is convinced.

No one else is changing; no one had been in the mini waiting room, either. I exit the door and begin to walk down the hall, but realize that I cannot remember which way to go. I feel disoriented and more vacuous than usual. I walk beneath the EXIT sign without seeing it. I overhear talking and the word "axilla."

All the nurses and Dr. Fi are gathered in the control room going over my paperwork. One of them spots me and they all look up; the conversation ends abruptly.

"Are you lost, darlin'?"

I have to think a moment, then answer with all sincerity, "I'm not sure. Am I?"

"Darlin', if you're *here*, you're lost." She walks me to the exit. On the way I see that the lights are shut off in the exam rooms. Full, tied-off trash bags have already been set out for the janitors. I am the last patient. I exit the hall into the lobby; empty. Even Dee is gone.

I drive home with a dull ringing in my ears, feeling more than slightly dingy, light-headed, yet above all else, oddly mellow. I do not know whether this is a physical side effect of the radiation, or perhaps a psychic effect, an absorption of spiritual energy from a place where so many patients face death and the big machines meant to burn it out of us. In any event, the noise of the day seems to have fallen away, leaving only the here and now.

I pull into the neighborhood and up to my driveway. A black sedan with tinted windows is parked in the driveway—a guest? But I do not recognize the car, and nobody else should be home right now. A robber? Who is this? I pull up directly behind the sedan, blocking it in. I will walk to the driver's door and get my explanation. But the sedan's back-up lights come on before I can exit Little Blue. The sedan backs toward me as I honk, long and loud, but it just keeps coming. Dammit. If it were any car but Little Blue I'd just take the hit to the front bumper, but The Penguin is in the shop and I need this car and don't want it wrecked. I back up hurriedly, just ahead of the black sedan. It turns away and tears off down the road.

This is odd, not to mention disturbing. Death drives an Altima? I hustle into the house—it has not been robbed. I call Jenelle and tell her of the black car and all its possible implications. Her reaction is such that I can nearly see the rolling of her eyes on the other end of the phone. I want her to empathize, but I let it go, water off a duck's back, for today is a beautiful day. I've been irradiated and I'm ready to glow in the dark if need be. It is a done deal. I have been treated; the MDA decision is off my plate. Tomorrow I will learn about my own chemotherapy. F_ _ _ cancer!

I catch a glimpse of myself in the bathroom mirror. A diamond pattern is embossed clearly into my forehead. F _ _ _ that damned mask, too!

Later, I find a large sky-blue Post-It note on my desk and fill in the following entry:

1/10/08, 10:28 PM, NOTE FOR FILE: I feel ever so slightly dizzy, strangely mellow. Still worried about stomach.

Chemoteach

I arrive at 10:50 for my 11:15 a.m. appointment The parking situation is atrocious; apparently the cancer business is good.

Chemo patients have no special parking spots, so I am obliged to park in the south forty and walk in the bright sunlight, which I was told the day before not to do during radiation treatment.

I sit in the waiting room of Dr. X. This also happens to be the same waiting room for people going to chemotherapy, and for those of us learning about chemotherapy. Jenelle shows up, straight from work. I like it when she comes to appointments—it feels like I'm not so all alone against this demon.

I get called in a bit early, not to see Dr. X or the chemotherapy nurse, but to have a conversation with a speakerphone. There is a private office for doing this, and I sit at a desk and stare at the phone. I don't know the purpose of this until the phone comes to life.

The call is with a "business office specialist" for the cancer center. She reviews my healthcare coverage: "Your insurance company will pay zero percent and you will pay one hundred percent until the $3,000 deductible is reached. At that point, the insurance company will pay eighty percent and you will pay twenty percent until your out-of-pocket total reaches $8,000, at which point the insurance company will pay one hundred percent."

I recall that our deductible started anew on New Year's. "Whoa, whoa, whoa," I protest, "how can it be possible that I have to pay the first $3,000 and they pay nothing?"

"Because that's your coverage."

"But what can I do about that?"

"I would advise that you get better insurance."

There is no real negotiating going on—only informing the patient, me, of my obligation. I say, "How much of the $3,000 deductible do I have left?"

"Hold on...Uhm, $2,825 left on your deductible. Will you be paying cash or credit card?" I agree to load up a credit card, and foresee it filling up to $8,000 rapidly.

Due to my prior good health, I had no idea how much deductible and out-of-pocket cash was involved in big-ticket hobbies such as cancer. We have decent financial resources in our household; I wonder how people with average or below-average incomes handle it. I suppose that they must go broke.

I am sent back out to the waiting room to further ponder monthly cash flow. Hmm...we just bought a house and spent all our liquid assets... we're paying for Carina's tuition... therefore, I have no idea where I am going to come up with $8,000. Maybe I can sell something! Jenelle's car? I glance over at her. She reads a paperback and looks peaceful enough right now, but if I tried to sell her car, she'd kill me. Carina's car? No, that would also get me killed by Jenelle. One of my two cars? No... might as well kill myself. Hmm. I ponder a while longer, but feel backed into a corner. I decide to take one for the team and sell Little Blue. She's a sweet ride, but she's fully paid-for and eight grand is eight grand. Hell of a way to start the day.

We get called back in by a woman perhaps ten years my senior. "Hi," she says, "I'm Nurse Gentle, your chemotherapy nurse."

Wow, I think, I have a chemotherapy nurse! This cancer thing is like a Cecil B. DeMille flick with a cast of thousands.

Jenelle and I introduce ourselves to Nurse Gentle, and we work our way back to a small office with a window to the hallway (open, no blinds) and a window to the outside world (blinds drawn). The floor of the office is perhaps ten feet on a side. There is a comfy chair—La-Z-Boy style—for the victim, and a chair that looks to be of medium comfort for a companion. That would be for Jenelle.

Nurse Gentle jumps right into the chemical itinerary. I whip out the notebook and begin to write furiously, and Jenelle does the same.

"You will receive two chemos, twenty-one days apart, with a possible third chemo depending on how the first two go. Your chemo will be Ethyol in conjunction with Cisplatin, bought under the "Platinol" trade name. No portacath is indicated at this time. Most of the side effects are reversible. In your case you will have less of a dose *than some*, and so should have fewer side effects *than some*. The nausea and vomiting will likely only last a week or so, and by the way, you need to make sure you have your anti-nausea prescription ready beforehand.

"Your nadir, or lowest point in your blood counts, will occur ten days after treatment, and your counts will not return to normal until perhaps fourteen to twenty days after treatment. You must drink water and lots of it—I cannot overemphasize this point, as it helps prevent some of the kidney damage you will sustain. You must eat regular meals, and eat them on time regardless of hunger level."

"Uhm, excuse me," I say, trying to work a word in edgewise. "Will I need to have any sort of special diet?"

"Eat and drink as normal, but watch out for dehydration, especially with caffeine."

"Will I lose my hair?"

"Maybe. It's not a large dose. Some people do, and some don't with this level. If so, it will be a couple of weeks after treatment. I can guarantee that you will have some thinning. There is one very important point that I must make. Do not—I repeat—do not impregnate your wife at this time." I look over at Jenelle and she at me. We both laugh—this is the last thing either of us want.

"Aside from not impregnating your wife, it is important that you do not take aspirin. Here are the numbers for the clinic and for me in the event that you get shaking chills or uncontrolled vomiting." She hands me a card with the phone numbers. "Drink two to three quarts of water every twenty four-hours. Avoid crowds. Wash your hands, wash your hands, wash your hands! Minimize or eliminate alcohol."

"Not even a glass of wine with dinner?"

"Trust me, you won't want a drink and if you have one, it will likely make you nauseous."

"I believe you, but I *already* want a drink."

"Avoid sun exposure. Bananas are good. Eat a plain old nutritious diet. I'll need your CBC before your second treatment."

"CBC?" I say.

"Complete Blood Count. Also, report symptoms such as numbness and tingling. Now, back to the Ethyol," she says. "This is a protectant drug that mitigates side effects of the Cisplatin. We give it to you prior. You have to drink plenty of fluids—the chemo causes low blood pressure and can cause severe nausea. By the way, bring your lunch to chemo, it lasts a full shift, basically all day. Show up at 8:30 AM. Now, once you go home again, be sure and call the doctor if your fever goes over one-hundred degrees, or if you have a tremendous amount of vomiting. If you have radiation scheduled for that day, call them and let them know, and they'll make sure you don't have to wait too long. Hmm, I think that's about it. Any questions?"

"Can a person sprain their hand from writing too fast?"

"No," she says.

"Okay," I say, "I'm good."

January 14

It is Monday, and I await radiation treatment number three. There is no radiation on weekends, as The Beast, the nurses, the doctors, and everyone except Lumpy take days off. (That's when Lumpy does pushups.) The waiting room holds several sickly looking individuals and one strapping guy about my age. I want to ask him what he's in for, but Nurse WW calls me before I get the chance.

My head is bolted to the slab and The Beast rotates and buzzes through its stations. I find myself blocking it all out, hoping I can fast-forward to the end of radiation number thirty. As I lay here, I again ponder the others enduring this treatment. People on this machine are stripped of the illusions that most of us like to shield ourselves with in daily life. We are forced to confront reality, and reality is raw and harsh. I am at the mercy of a giant, one-eyed emotionless robot. I pray; we all pray.

I drive home alone—mellow, ditzy, tired.

Doc Skin calls. He has finally spoken with the formerly unavailable Dr. Gone. They have studied my files. Dr. Gone says no squamous-cell skin cancers were ever removed, especially from Lumpy's vicinity. Doc Skin has discussed my case with one of his buddies at the Mayo Clinic who believes it's a stretch to think that a squamous-cell skin cancer not in the immediate proximity of Lumpy could have caused this. Yet the two of them feel that there still could be a skin-cancer connection.

The phone call is thirteen-minutes long and by the end of it, I am convinced that Doc Skin finds my case to be a cool mystery to be solved: C.S.I. Armpit. Whatever it takes to turn him on, I'm on board.

January 15: Chemo Day

Journal entry, 6:30 AM:

Beware the Ides of January. Today I expose my irradiated but otherwise pure body to perhaps a half dozen drugs, one more corrosive than the rest: Cisplatin. I've been mellow, upset, sad, glad, happy, depressed, the whole gamut lately. Yesterday I went in early to work (got up at 4:45 AM). I was at my desk by 5:50 AM. I went to the gym near work. I did a 10-minute, level 12 regimen. No problem, but my lungs seemed to wheeze a bit. It seems like I read that happens during radiation, but I cannot remember.

Jenelle accompanies me to the cancer center. I wear comfy clothes (a tee shirt, sweat pants, tennis shoes), and look like I am going to a sleepover. In the waiting room the TV blares local news—one of the worst audio-visual assaults I have been forced to endure thus far.

"*Blah, blah, terror! Early female puberty! Pirates! What's in your refrigerator can kill you!*"   Local TV news is brain junk food – like cheese fries covered in sausage gravy, wrapped in a Twinkie, supersized and mainlined with high fructose corn syrup and a side order of lobotomy. At this moment, nobody else in the waiting room watches—they stare out, talk, read. How do they do it? I cannot *not* hear the damn TV.

So many lucky old people! Sure, they're cancer patients and all, but they did make it to old age. Will I? How do these old-timers manage to ignore the TV? Is that their secret?

I am called up to the reception desk. Job one: Show ID. Job two: Give away money. J's medical MasterCard is declined. Twice. I am about to endure chemotherapy *and* I have to pay $2,825 on my personal Visa. It occurs to me that doctors used to file insurance first and bill the patient later, but to be fair I suppose it's difficult to collect from people who might die, or even think that they might die, so they get it upfront. This, I decide, is sound business practice, and hand over the card.

The news about pirates continues after an ad for prescription blood-pressure medicine ("Ask for it by name."). We are called in by Nurse Gentle as Lumpy and his crew hoist the Jolly Roger, prepare swords, and ready the grappling hooks. They won't be caught unawares.

I get to choose which room to take chemo in. I see a few private suites which are no larger than closets, and one grand room filled with La-Z-Boys and IV racks for steerage class. Jenelle's insurance, expensive and filled with obscene deductibles as it is, apparently pays closet class. I pick the one where we did Chemoteach.

I open the blind for some lovely ambient light, as I want to enjoy each living moment in the beautiful world around me, even on Chemo Day. A couple with children strolls past on the sidewalk a few feet away from me; they stare into the chemo closet. Beyond them I see a parking lot filled with pickup trucks and SUVs, then a freeway filled with pickup trucks and SUVs. I close the blind. Jenelle fires up her laptop.

Nurse Gentle comes in carrying a plastic needle-like device with a tube hanging off one end. "Which hand do you want it in?" she says.

Yours, I think. But I say: "I'm feeling left-brained, so use the right."

She does not appear to appreciate my clever banter and proceeds to lay a blue paper towel on my right wrist. She applies a tourniquet, then swabs my forearm a few inches above that.

Holding the paper towel in one hand and the needle in the other, Nurse Gentle is now all out of hands. So she uncaps the tube with her mouth. She then jams the needle into the chosen vein. I ponder the sanitary implications of the mouth method of handling chemo, but say nothing. I do not want to piss her off as she is the one holding the needle.

There is a lot of blood. This whole episode is noticeably messier than the drawing of samples upstairs in the lab. None of my life juice gets on the La-Z-Boy, however. Nurse Gentle's towels and caps and bits and bobs almost fall off of the arm of my chair, and I do not feel reassured. But before you know it, I look down and see that a quick-disconnect fitting has been installed into my arm, strapped down with sturdy-looking medical tape. All the various chemicals and poisons will pass through this tube over the course of the day. It won't move because it is taped securely to my arm hair. I take a picture with my cell phone.

We have now been here fifty minutes, and all I've done so far is pay $2,825 for a messy needle installation. It is 9:20 AM, and we await The Mix. There is a kitchen somewhere (in a hollow tree, I presume), and medical technicians are running around there in chef's hats, whipping up batches of chemicals for all the La-Z-Boy squatters. I'm told that my special brew is not ready just yet; perhaps one of the elves had to go out for paprika. Jenelle works on a spreadsheet while I write in my cancer journal and read car magazines.

The door to my luxury closet is open; nurses and patients wander by with IVs and clipboards. I am supposed to drink plenty of water, so I've have been hydrating like a big dog. I always strive to be the best at what I do, and have been to the restroom twice already. I might go again. My secret is imagining that the bottled water is beer.

I take more phone pictures of my arm and of the room, and ask Jenelle to take one of me. She does, while proclaiming me "goofy." In Jenelle's photo I look high as a kite, although I have not had a drop of chemicals yet.

The Mix

The Mix arrives. Nurse Gentle hangs four bags on the IV pole and hooks one up. It is Aloxi, and feels cool going in. The bags are the size of McDonald's French fry bags. It should be noted that, this time, Nurse Gentle produces a pair of nitrile gloves prior to handling my fitting or any chemicals. One of her gloves nearly drops to the floor; but agile Nurse Gentle scoops it up before it hits (at least I think it's before). She slips it on.

The next drug is Ranitidine. "For the tummy," she announces. Ranitidine feels cool going in as well. I wonder if it will make me randy. This does not happen, and the drug runs out at 9:52 AM. I watch as the last drops go into my vein. Nurse Gentle is nowhere in sight. Next I watch as blood goes back up the hose toward the bag. Nurse Gentle remains nowhere in sight.

"Jenelle," I say. No response. She is absorbed in a particularly engrossing email. "Uhm, blood!" I exclaim. "Wrong way! Not good!"

Jenelle looks at the hose, then jumps up and fetches Nurse Gentle's assistant, Nurse GA, who runs in and turns off the Ranitidine. The reverse blood flow stops. I chalk that one up to Amusing Chemo Surprises and prepare myself to move on.

"What's next?" I say.

"Dexameth—a steroid," Nurse GA informs me.

I ponder talking like Arnold Schwarzenegger, think better of it, then go ahead. "Vhat ees de puhpuss off dis stay-roid with vich you vill *pump me up*?"

She is not amused, yet answers anyway: "It averts an allergic reaction to the chemo," she says. "The side effects are hunger, a red face, and waking up at the witching hour."

"I have all that anyway."

At 10:17 AM, Ativan goes in. This is supposed to make me sleepy and calm. Before long, this theory is proven correct.

At 10:25 AM, the first *big* bag gets hung up. It is a voluptuous sack of saline solution with potassium and magnesium mixed in. This is supposed to hydrate me even more and might take two hours to drain into me. I nap.

At 1:05 PM I awaken, groggy and placid. Nurse Gentle enters and hangs up the big boy: The Cisplatin, or as I like to call it, Cislumpypoison. Before connecting the hose, she gives me the "Ethyol push."

While hooking up the Ethyol she says, "Oh, by the way, some people have a reaction."

"What sort of reaction?"

"Well, you might need this." She hands me what appears to be a condom for the world's most well-hung race horse.

"Are you telling me that this IV is filled with bionic Viagra?"

"No," she says, with a disapproving schoolmarm look, "this is a barf bag. Some people become violently ill and throw up all over the place."

I nod knowingly while watching the chemical enter my vein. "And how long does that usually take?"

She looks at her watch. "You're safe. You'd be puking by now." She looks over at the equine porn-star condom. "Better save that just in case, though."

"For the puking, you mean."

"Yeah. For the puking."

At 1:26 PM, the Cisplatin enters my veins to seek out and destroy fast-dividing cells, which include blood cells, hair follicles, cells of the mouth, and all other collateral damage (kill 'em all! let God sort 'em out!). I hope that Lumpy will be amongst the casualties. I do not puke, nor does any of my anatomy become the size and shape required to fill the horse prophylactic. I detect no immediate reaction. I ponder weapons of medical mass destruction while drifting back to sleep.

At 3:00 PM, I remain mellow. Nurse Gentle arrives with a pair of Livestrong bracelets. I am still tapped into the last of the Cisplatin on my right side, so I put Livestrong on my left wrist. Jenelle puts hers on her right. If I wasn't in the club before, I sure as hell am now. I have toxic chemicals coursing through my veins, I am radioactive, and most of all, I have earned a Livestrong bracelet—the hard way.

I get up to pee again, but before I go, I have Jenelle take another picture of me. I am virile, strong, filled with chemicals, and groggy as hell.

"I'm taking this IV pole with us!" I say. "We paid twenty-eight hundred and twenty-five dollars for it."

6 A KILLING ROUTINE

Morning journal entry, January 17, 2008:

I am alive. I'm not nauseous. I feel pretty well, as a matter of fact. I've felt worse on non-cancer days (self-inflicted hangovers).

I feel a bit loopy and my coffee tastes funny. I'm cautiously optimistic about my physical condition, but understand that Cisplatin is poison and does its work over time. I intend to work and unless something odd happens, I won't be bedridden. My system feels like the downside of a drunk: Shagged out with no remaining buzz.

I want to rebel and continue exercising, but can't decide whether to wait until tomorrow, as I fear sweating out my dose of chemo. Nobody has warned me that this is even possible, but what if I can? I have a stomachache at the moment and continue to have a dull discomfort along the left side, where my ribs meet my gut.

I am not unaffected mentally. There is some brain fuzz; there are mood swings. I cried at supper last night. I'd been telling Jenelle about various cancer patients I've met, two of whom had completed treatment only to have their wives diagnosed with breast cancer afterward. And that's a small sample set, statistically speaking. But the thing is, I don't think I was particularly swayed by those stories so much as feeling a need to cry. I feel out of kilter, off balance, hazy. Manic depression is a frustrating mess.

Ok, I can't stay away from the gym due to my Lance-like exercise mania. I work ten minutes at level twelve on the escalator stair machine, plus legs, then stretch and work abs and lower back. I feel good physically, but even after the workout, my brain remains blurred.

In the locker room, I suddenly feel odd aches throughout my body, and find myself linking all physical symptoms to cancer. It's all cancer. On that note, I drive to the cancer center.

Journal entries:

10:45 AM: Walked up to give blood for CBC.

11:05 AM: Was called to the back for blood work—more forms to sign and initial—the nurse (got a new one) complimented me on my veins.

11:20 AM: Walked to lobby of hospital to ask about getting my pathology slides (from Doc Young's biopsy). I asked the helper at the main information desk where to go, & he looked at me like I was insane. He said, "I don't know, try Medical Information Technology." I said, "How about the lab?" He said, "No, try Medical Information Technology." I went there. They sent me to the lab.

The employees (one woman & one man) at the lab were picking at each other, fighting like brother & sister—goofing around, & generally acting like clowns. The woman got her boss. Boss Lady One heard my request & went to ask the next higher boss (Boss Lady Two). Boss Lady One returned & said they'd have to order the slides. I filled out a form and turned it into the goofy woman.

11:30 AM: Walked over for chest X-ray.

NOTE: TV blares; one old guy out of 12 people in waiting room watches. TVs blare in every freaking waiting room every time—most often on TV news. I turn them off whenever possible.

I just remembered, I told Dr. X of my dull ache on my LHS (@ ribcage). She blew it off as stress-related. I hope she's right.

By 11:54 AM, the old guy who had been watching TV has left. I am called to a desk to fill out more paperwork. The clerk asks which doctor sent me here. I tell him Dr. X.

"Not Dr. The Man?"

"No, it's for Dr. X."

He prints me an ID bracelet and places it on my wrist. I return to my seat and look at my tag. It says "Dr. The Man."

I get a chest X-ray, but according to the technician, because of the combination of the shape of my torso and lungs, and the size of the X-ray target, she needs to take two X-rays. I figure she doesn't know what the hell she's doing. I also figure that I have now received more radiation that will give me yet more cancer. But then compared to The Beast, X-rays are like pissing in the ocean.

I wander to the radiation waiting room for a follow-up consultation with Dr. Fi. While I leaf through a cancer magazine (*Cauliflower Doesn't Have to be Boring!; Bladder Cancer—One Wife's Story*), a man sits down across from me. He says nothing so I introduce myself. He tells me his name is Hubert. Hubert is a sad sack, woe-is-me sort. He carps a lot and comes across as generally despondent and depressed. He complains of fatigue. I ask him if he has a mesh mask to hold his head down, and he says no. I ask where his radiation is applied, and he motions across his belly and rolls his eyes. Nurse One calls me back to see Dr. Fi. I say bye to Hubert, but he does not reply.

I am put into an exam room and then left alone. I play with the electric adjustments for the chair, and while in a reclined position, try to hook myself up to the blood-pressure machine. Dr. Fi. is to meet me once a week to hear my concerns and questions, bad jokes and mortal fears. Luckily she shows up when I'm taking a break from medical equipment mischief.

"Any questions?" she asks.

"Yes. Can I get a spare mesh face mask for home use?"

At first she seems baffled, then seems to understand that it's a joke. "And what use do you have in mind?" she says, eyebrows raised.

I raise my eyebrows twice in return, and she laughs. It never gets old, making cancer professionals laugh.

I mention to Dr. Fi that I see a lot of swelling in my left shoulder. She has me yank my shirt up and looks me over, then asks if I am right-handed. I say yes.

"Do you do anything with your left hand?" There's an obvious comeback, but I restrain myself.

"Sometimes I use my computer mouse with my left hand."

"Why would you do such a thing?"

"That's how my mouse rolls."

She explains how physical activity on the radiation side can lead to extra swelling, and working a mouse apparently counts as activity. I wonder if Lumpy is swollen. I wonder if Lumpy will pop.

She finishes with me and, as I put my shirt on, I hear Hubert being led in for his post-zap Q&A period, one exam room over. While I walk toward the waiting room, Dr. Fi asks Hubert how he is doing.

"Oh, I don't know," he sighs. "I don't know if I'm making any progress. Maybe you can tell me if I'm okay." All this in that sad-sack voice.

I have heard that, for cancer survival, attitude is key and optimism crucial. If so, Hubert is screwed. Now watch him outlive us all....

* * *

As Jenelle cooks, I mention a craving for gooey cookies. Usually I don't crave sweets, but chemo does odd things. She whips up a batch of chocolate chip cookies, and serves them still warm with vanilla ice cream. They taste pretty good, but each serving leaves a bitter taste in my mouth. Not a huge turn-off, but still unpleasant. Food has already lost a bit of its flavor—say, one-quarter to one-third of its taste—which is still not bad compared to stories I have heard.

I drive to the taekwondo school to pick Kaily up after class. On the way over I feel myself lapsing into exhaustion. I want to be my normal self, but barely manage to poke my head in the door to say hi to Master Steel Curtain.

Suddenly I feel ashamed of being in a fog, feeling depressed, not being in class, having cancer. I don't even have the drive to say "F _ _ _ cancer!" or even "Foreplay cancer!" I just want to lie down. I hope that all of my days will not be like this one. Cancer is a full-time freaking second job. I feel utterly Hubertesque.

Tonight Mom and Dad come to our house to celebrate my birthday. A good son would rejoice and be thankful for familial love. A good son would anxiously await his good parents. What I want to do is take a nap, then leave town before they show up.

I love Mom and Dad, and it's great that I receive an outpouring of love and concern, but the *phone calls*. Not just from Mom and Dad, but from every-freaking-body. It's a bad case of triple-C (Concerned Cancer Communications). These had calmed down after my Christmas email, but now they're back with a vengeance. I barely have time to make it to the doctor, work, exercise and eat and sleep, and answer emails. I end up telling my story over and over. My brother Bryan called yesterday when I got back from Dr. Otherdermo, and talked for a half hour. Now, Mom and Dad will be here in person. Oh, they will be supportive. They will also want to know about what I am going through while not talking about it, i.e., the Heavy Topic Paradox.

I won't tell my parents about my secret desire to be left alone, because then they won't think that I'm the good son (although they may not have thought that since I was eleven). Cancer is turning out to be quite vexing from a purely selfish perspective. I want it all: I want to be loved and cared for, *and* I want everyone to leave me the hell alone. Sometimes I want to not answer other people's questions when I have so many myself. I want to sit atop a grassy knoll and ask the sunset: "Will I die?"

"Yes my son," intones the dusk, "but I will not tell you when."

* * *

Happy 44th birthday! I am still here. In the mirror I notice a loose eyelash. I reach up and grab it, and four more come out with it. For a present to myself, I won't go to radiation today. Actually, it is Saturday and there is no radiation anyway. Good timing for a birthday.

* * *

Mom and Dad have gone and I go to work around 6:00 AM. I am alone in the office with Armchair. At around 6:45 he asks me about the side effects from chemo. I tell the story of the loose eyelashes on my birthday. As I speak, I grab a bit of hair on the top of my head and give it a light tug between thumb and forefinger.

"I'm not sure when I'll start losing this hair." Then I look at my fingers and see a few hairs in my grasp. "Oh, right now, I guess."

I visit the gym at lunchtime. I perform well on the escalator stair machine while reading *In Cold Blood* for ten minutes. I work my legs and stretch. I feel good.

At 3:00 I drive home via the cancer center so I can pick up my pathology slides. The nurse does not know what to do, so she asks a Boss Lady behind the scenes.

Boss Lady yells, "Who's it for?"

The nurse asks, "Who's it for?"

I say "Baskett."

The nurse yells, "Baskett!"

Boss Lady shouts, "They're right there!"

"Right where?"

"The only Baskett there!"

The nurse looks down and grabs the solitary envelope. "Baskett" is written on it, large in Magic Marker. She hands it to me with no ID check, no nada. Cancer imposters could have a field day with these people.

January 22

I keep finding bits of loose hair—not much, just a few hairs here or there around my head. I could get upset about this but prefer the opposite tack: I am pleased, ecstatic almost, as dead hairs mean dead cancer cells. Screw the cancer! Kill it! Destroy! We are beyond cosmetic concerns at this point.

I check in for radiation and sit across from Hubert, who says nothing. I've already read the current issue of the cancer magazine (*Amazing Realism In Nose Prosthetics*; *How Much of my Colon Can I Live Without?*). Nurse Wonder Woman calls me back and I don the gown. I lay on the sheet while she bolts me down via mesh face mask. The steel slab feels especially cold and hard today.

There comes a moment where the only noise I hear is whirring cooling fans—the closest thing to silence in the radiation chamber. I stare into the eye of The Beast, lifeless and inanimate. I have no choice but to trust that this radiating monster will not come unleashed and turn on me, first vaporizing me and then the staff at the onset of its rampage across the city, melting tanks and exploding fighter planes with its hellish death rays. How diligent were the programmers who choreographed its dance? How sane were the scientists and engineers who designed its motors and radiation gates, and delineated the precision of its aim?

The Beast's head suddenly comes to life and traverses around me, exposing the peaceful landscape scene built into the ceiling. This time I remain obsessed with The Beast itself and fail to embrace the odd spirituality of the place. The head stops at Station one out of my range of vision. By Station three I can see into its eye. The microwave hum begins and I count steamboats. The interlaced bars that form the iris of The Beast normally shift into position before the zap begins. However, as I glance up, I notice that they are moving *during* the zap.

I jerk involuntarily against the mesh face mask—have I just pulled a muscle in my neck? There's been a malfunction! Oh my God! I'm trapped!

What if I'm wrong and it's not a malfunction? But what if it is? I dare not move, or I'll cook something I don't want cooked. Despite the panic, I haven't moved out of my Underwear Model Pose; my right hand still grips the cold stainless-steel rail.

Close your eyes, I tell myself. *Breathe in.* I must be mistaken. I don't want to be a big baby or make a scene, but also I don't want random radiation strewn about all over the place, baking my gizzards. What do I do? Call out? I can't even move my freaking mouth. It must be okay; The Beast is a high-tech marvel. But the shutters never did that before! I am mentally paralyzed and forced to trust more than I'm accustomed to. I do nothing, say nothing. "They" must know what "they" are doing.

I remain on high alert, listening for odd sounds, watching for other odd movements out of the corner of my eye until finally the slab drops and The Beast's head ramps back over the top of me and goes to sleep at last. Nurse One appears in my field of vision.

"Well, there, partner! Another one gone!" She unbolts my face from the steel slab. I say nothing. "Are ya all right, darlin'?"

I just sit up and leave.

Afterward, I can find no one of authority to whom I can report this aberration. I don't trust the nurses with information of malfunctions for fear that will pop the Beast's hood and whip out the hammer. I'll call Dr. Fi when I get home, and let her know.

F-ing abject panic! F_ _ _ cancer! Die Lumpy, you son of a bitch. But leave me out of it!

Dr. Fi calls back about a half hour later, after I've left a lengthy, panicked voicemail on the cancer center phone system.

"Relax," she says, "those shutters are supposed to move as the radiation is applied."

"Then how come I've never noticed this before?"

"Perhaps you have, but you do not remember."

"No way, my memory is...." There comes a pause.

"Yes?"

"Good point," I say. "Maybe I forgot or just never noticed."

"Relax. There is constant feedback on the exact position of the head and the shutters and all aspects of the radiation treatment. If anything went wrong with that machine we would know immediately and it would shut itself down."

"But what about—"

"Relax. I seem to recall that you are an engineer."

"Yeah I'm an engineer, but the machine—"

"Relax. This sort of thing happens now and then with engineers."

Last week of January

My throat begins to hurt a bit more each day; now it is ongoing and annoying on the left side. I need to ask Dr. Fi if this is okay.

On the bright side, I'm one-third finished with radiation; ten of thirty zap sessions are in the can.

I speak with Ken, a fellow radiation patient (non-Hodgkin's Lymphoma) who has also completed ten of thirty treatments; he usually goes under The Beast right before me. He sells medical equipment across a fair-sized territory that stretches from Houston to College Station, where fanatical Aggies are trained. Ken lives north of town near an MD Anderson satellite facility, yet comes to our cancer center. He knows lots of doctors of various specialties who agree that Dr. The Man is in fact THE MAN. This I like.

"How's your relationship with your wife?" Ken says.

"Fine, why do you ask?"

"Cancer," he intones, "either brings a marriage closer together or splits it apart."

So far it has only brought Jenelle and me closer together. Hasn't it? Oh sure, our Norman Rockwell look has seemed misleading over the years (unless Norman used to also paint epic battle scenes), and marriage tests the souls of all involved, but my wife and I have leapt into the fray together to kill Lumpy, and any problems from the past are forgotten. There is only now.

* * *

The weather is dreary. Jenelle's job has taken her offshore while the floor people have arrived to rip up the carpet and level the floor for maple. My throat hurts like hell. Part of me feels woefully lonely and abandoned, but I stuff that inside and tamp it down. And life is not all bad because I've completed eleven of thirty radiations, and I get to work from home until the end of next week due to white-cell nadir. When I can fight off feeling abandoned I remain upbeat and in a good mood—that is until night, at which time I crash from a pervasive lack of energy, lie down, and feel sorry for myself.

The weather turns nice for the weekend, but I am supposed to avoid the sun during radiation and chemo. There are always windows to gaze through. Jenelle remains offshore in the Gulf and sends an email informing me I'll spend one more night alone in bed.

* * *

Journal entry:

I had odd dreams last night. Violent and ugly. I'll just assume that I was subconsciously dispatching cancer that had appeared in the form of a man.

I walk like Shaggy from Scooby Doo sometimes. Not intentionally, but as a result of my brain-damaged state. I feel more odd this morning than usual. Sort of dizzy. Well, not quite dizzy, but verging in that direction.

The floor dudes finish laying maple planks. Good *feng shui* transforms the room and adds a positive energy to the house. I need this sort of beauty and calming influence. I continue to obsess about cars. Even more than B.C. (Before Cancer), Craig's List has become an addiction. Maybe this feeling will subside once I get The Penguin back. But I always need one more hit....

I drive to the taekwondo school during the workday when nobody else is around and kick the "mean guy" dummy and the heavy bag. It feels extra good in that magnified way I seem to be feeling things lately, good as well as bad. Everything is at 110%. I am beginning to fall in love with life and living it well, Lumpy be damned.

I work hard on a Firm D project, doubling up on my effort because I felt too weird to work yesterday. I don't quit until 10:30 PM. I probably shouldn't do this, especially on Nadir Day. But maybe if I pretend hard enough that I'm well, then everything will be okay.

* * *

By 5:30 tonight I will have finished my halfway point in radiation. My skin is becoming dry and irritated on the cancer side, and the same shoulder becomes achy quite easily—it cannot stand much use, or even sleeping on it, which sucks because that's the side I like to sleep on.

I can still feel a hard mass under my left armpit but it does seem that Lumpy has shrunk a little. Whether this is just reduced post-surgical swelling or the healing of scar tissue, who knows? In any event, that slimy death bastard is smaller. Me likey.

Today there are two newbies in radiation: an older dude (fifty-plus), who looks like Joe Suburbia from Peoria—his wife brought him—and a black woman who is not a newbie, as she has a wig on. She acts quite shy and doesn't say a thing; she looks down a lot. I've had days like that.

Ken is here. He tells me that he's the worst patient ever—doesn't listen to any of his dietary advice, pushes himself at work. He even skipped his radiation a couple days ago to go to a business dinner with his out-of-town boss. I read between the lines that Ken's boss doesn't know that Ken has cancer. I can relate; it makes me less upset if I keep pretending to have a normal life.

I did push it yesterday at work, but I would never skip treatment for work reasons, therefore I am not as obsessed with being normal as Ken, right? I am in denial about being in denial. Zap! Drive. Eat. Sleep, wake up. Repeat.

* * *

Firm D has a big deadline. I put in high-intensity hours, even though I'm far from 100%. My plan for living well is in conflict with itself, as I am supposed to stop and smell the roses, as well as keep a job and be normal. *Normal* seems to be winning out lately, while the smelling of roses sucks hind teat. Will the rush end? Can it? Not unless something changes.

I take out an ad for Little Blue on Craig's List; a man from Colorado calls about her. His offer stands at $800 less than my asking price. I call him back and split the difference. Done deal. Maybe now I'll be able to clear out some of these medical bills. But I'll miss that little death-race toy.

7 NADIR HIJINKS

It's not that I consider them inherently evil, these people. I'm trying to be more understanding these days, embrace my fellow man and have empathy for their suffering—we're all in this armpit together. However, I am moody and they are my enemies; I see through their disguises.

Look at that one over there. Beauty-parlor hair and polyester pants and oversized bifocals. Oh, don't sneeze, grandma! No! You white prune, you did that on purpose!

Am I being paranoid? Or just careful? You see, if my resistance to infection is so compromised by dipping blood-cell counts that I'm being advised to avoid public places, then what's the one public place I should avoid at all costs? Answer: a waiting room populated by Typhoid Mary's grandmother. I know she's sick—why else would she be sneezing in a blood lab?

Cancer Club members should have secret side entrances to our own waiting rooms, preferably with sliding peepholes, and hale and hearty bouncers:

"Can I help youse?"

"Dr. Fi sent me."

"What's da password?"

"Stage four needle chemo lump."

"Okay, Mac, c'mon in."

But the system is flawed and it doesn't work that way. Today there are four infected enemy combatants, all spread out to keep me from sitting a safe distance away. A newspaper lowers and I realize that one of the four is a fellow club member, Ken, who awaits his own CBC. We exchange greetings and a few cancer vocabulary words and acronyms. Ken gets called in right away, leaving three more virus carriers ahead of me.

There is one girl working the whole place. She doesn't look up from her paperwork. I announce that I'm here for my CBC. She still doesn't look up but she mutters, "Please take a seat and I'll be with you shortly."

Now comes the Herd. Grandma must have given the secret signal, because people stream in like there's a free pancake breakfast and drop their paperwork in the basket. I've got no paperwork because my CBC is a standing order. Time passes. I'm not getting called. Yet more reinforcements stream in.

Amongst the rabble, two women have wet, phlegmy coughs. What the hell? One sits right freaking, beside me! Oh, you *are* inherently evil. What's scarier at this moment, catching pneumonia off of Betty Bacteria, or looking rude and paranoid for jumping up and sprinting across the room? But who knows what microbes Marvin Mullet over there is packing? Strep gonads or maybe just an infection that makes him think it's still 1986.

And the TV blares. I have to violate my own principles and look up at it because I need an escape. In India, day laborers have been waking up in strange beds with sore backs and missing kidneys. Good God, hot robot news-reading chick, tell me more! The laborers were supposed to score lucrative jobs, but employment was a ruse perpetrated by a ring of organ thieves. Lick your lip gloss! Do it!

Normally I would find kidney thievery odd, even for a cable news story, but it makes me wonder: if there are customers for kidneys, how about other parts grown inside (such as Lumpy) for discerning shoppers on the outer fringe of kinky? "Kidney? Intriguing, but that's so last month. What else have you got? Oh, my! A tumor? Wrap it up, I'll take it to go!" How much would Lumpy be worth on the open market? Probably not much now that he's damaged.

I have to resign myself to the fact that sitting around a waiting room filled with the ill, who could be as much of a threat to me as an Indian tumor thief, has become the new normal. The initial shock of cancer has worn off, and I suppose that waking up one internal organ lighter wouldn't feel out of the ordinary at this point.

There are no seats left. The door swings open and another disease-ridden man arrives, bringing the total number of people in the waiting room to seventeen; this army believes in the Bush doctrine of shock and awe. The last infectious soldier announces to the receptionist that he has a standing order. She looks him up immediately and grabs a pile of papers out of the basket. She still doesn't call me.

Okay, this is freaking crazy! It's already 4:45, which happens to be my radiation appointment time. I swagger to the counter using my healthiest, manliest low-blood-count strut. "Hello!" I say, none too subtly.

"Oh!" the receptionist exclaims, startled by the combination of recognition and my psychotic demeanor. "You can go next!"

It's 4:50, I sit in the blood-drawing chair. "Busy out there," I say.

"You damn right!" my phlebotomist says. She looks up at the clock. "And if they think I'm stayin' a minute past five, they got another thing comin'!"

She mumbles a few more choice phrases under her breath and slams a drawer shut, then hastily slaps a tourniquet on my right arm. Fortunately, she nails the vein on the first try. She fidgets and taps her foot, watching one vial fill, and then the next, tossing them across the counter where they precariously roll back and forth. I stare at the vials, expecting them to smash upon the floor, painting the room red with my Lumpy-contaminated life fuel. But the samples come to rest and yet again I could have saved myself worry. I need to remember to let it go—all of it. It's just too bad I'm neurotic. Did cancer make me this way or is it a factory defect? No time for reflection now, I have a date with The Beast!

I hold my breath passing through the waiting room, by now surely teeming with cholera, consumption, contagious pregnancy. Without actually sprinting, I hit the stairs then pop out of the stairwell, practically running over Dr. The Man. Should I tell him about his flawed system? The missing peephole?

"Hello!" he says. "You're looking good. How are you?"

"I have a wicked case of pathogen paranoia, and those sick sons of bitches loitering around your waiting rooms are going to kill me before Lumpy can."

What I actually say is this: "Hi, Dr. The Man! I'm at my nadir, but doing pretty well, other than that."

"Excellent," he says, looking me over, "but keep that weight on!"

"What do you mean?"

"You're starting to make me look fat!"

"Umm...sure," I say. What's he talking about? I don't *feel* thin....

* * *

Farmer Ted is an old dude, late sixties I'd guess. He owns a truck with which he hauls freshly harvested Bermuda and St. Augustine grass all over Texas. His wife has breast cancer, and he drives her in everyday from outside of Brenham. He talks in that country wisdom way—unhurried and spare. He and I are trusting the system. We hope it works.

They are running late in radiation and so I manage to make my date with The Beast in plenty of time. In fact, they are running so late that Farmer Ted and I are able to kick back and have an in-depth conversation.

Farmer Ted tells me that he too had cancer, but that was a few years ago. He was a patient at MD Anderson. He now drinks beer, but at the time he wasn't allowed to because the cancer was in one of his kidneys. He suspects that he is still not allowed to drink beer, but doesn't ask in case they tell him so.

When I finally get called in for my zapping, Nurse One has me walk straight back to The Beast without putting on a gown. Nurse Two takes my picture for posterity (they take every victim's picture they tell me, even if they don't use the word "victim"). I shuck my shirt on the spot and lay down on The Beast. *Brr!*

February 1

I feel like I have a continual hangover, but without the headache or painful recollections of things I said that seemed appropriate at the time. I haven't exercised in several days. Also my inner engineer is grumpy: I was unable to review my blood counts yesterday afternoon at radiation as Dr. Fi was gone already by the time I arrived. I try to get my math fix by calculating how long we've been in our McMansion: two months. That seems too short; I count on my fingers twice to make sure. Okay, it's three months. Higher-math skills are definitely on the decline.

I arrive at the cancer center for yet another CBC—this one in preparation for my second round of chemo. The phlebotomist is a woman I haven't met before. She compliments me on my veins, which is usually a good sign. In fact, she finds my veins to be so fabulous that she tells me no tourniquet will be required. My ego feels soundly stroked as she goes straight for the jab. But she misses. She then proceeds to work the tip around in a sort of sewing-machine motion, withdraws it completely, and takes a big breath before jamming the whole needle into my arm up to the hilt—all manner of muscle and connective tissue are pierced, but no veins. Then she orders me to help apply the tourniquet on my left arm. "This should be a lesson to you," she scolds. "Don't let anyone do this without a tourniquet!"

Chemo II—The Sequel

Today is chemo day. I open a notification from Jenelle's insurance, informing me they are gracious enough to pay two thousand of the $9500 owed for my lymph-node surgery. Lovely. I suppose that J's insurance is better than nothing, but $7500 for the surgery plus all of the denied claims, plus a couple grand out of pocket for the first chemo—these are non-negligible figures! This I find stressful, even though I'll soon have money from selling Little Blue. Jenelle will come with me today. This I find comforting.

Nurse Gentle's assistant does me a favor and hooks up the valve in my left forearm so that I can take cell phone pictures with my right hand. I tell her how the hack phlebotomist butchered my right arm without a tourniquet.

"How could you let her do that?" she says.

"She threw me off my game by complimenting my blood vessels."

A few laughs, then Jenelle says, "You were thinking with the vein!" We all laugh harder—I think snot might come out of Nurse GA's nostrils.

We manage to land in the same purple office with the window overlooking the parking lot and highway, the room I had for my first round of chemo. I gaze with fondness upon the big La-Z-Boy. While I take a few phone pics, Jenelle settles down with a magazine. "You act like you're on vacation," she observes.

Nurse Gentle brings in a clear plastic tub of freshly brewed IV bags, hanging them on the rack, and then hooks me to the first one (anti-nausea). During the hookup, I observe little air bubbles passing through the clear plastic hose and entering my bloodstream. Some old memory of air bubbles in the blood being fatal, probably from '70s TV shows, urges me to declare an emergency. I say nothing, though, as Nurse Gentle appears quite unconcerned. I wonder if there has been some unannounced update of medical knowledge in the last few decades. The fluid is coolly slipping in, and I am not conking out from the air bubbles.

While I'm being lubed up, Jenelle makes a spreadsheet of medical claims to the tune of thousands of dollars. I begin to read *Strong Motion* by Jonathan Franzen. Good stuff—highly complex and interwoven, great details—and definitely hard to follow during chemotherapy. I need a book with more pictures.

Drug bag 2: Dexamethasone (a steroid). Nurse Gentle's assistant says I can play pro baseball after this. *Ha ha.*

Bag 3: Xantac (more anti-nausea)

Bag 4: Ativan (more anti-nausea—makes me sleepy)

Bag 5: Magnesium + Potassium

Bag 6: Manitol (unknown substance; possibly dissolves air bubbles in bloodstream). Shot after.

Bag 7: Ethyol (with horse condom)

Bag 8: Cisplatin. This is one big honking bag. I fall asleep.

The Bell

Nurse Gentle's assistant awakens me around 2:30. She reviews some papers and says, "Was that your last chemo?"

I have to think a moment. "Yeah. For now. We're supposed to re-evaluate later."

I stand in the doorway ready to check out and go take a nap, but she tells me to hold on. After disappearing she returns with a brass bell the size of a grapefruit.

"This," she says, "is the survivor bell."

Interesting, I think, but shrug my shoulders and undoubtedly look confused.

"It's a tradition I've had for years, and now it's a tradition at this hospital."

I stare a moment. "I'm not sure what this means," I say.

"It signals the end of chemo! You've survived!"

"You're giving it to me?"

"No, I'm not giving it *to* you! You ring it!"

"Oh! Cool!" But before I grab the bell, I pause to hear a voice inside my head: *If you ring this bell, you're a fraud. You only have entry-level cancer; those were only two chemo-light treatments.*

I'm no fraud! I've got Lumpy up my armpit, trying to kill me!

Other chemo patients are wondering why you're not bald. Don't ring it.

I realize that this has become an awkward moment—Nurse Gentle continues to hold up the bell and I stare at it like a doped-up Summer of Love participant, except that I don't feel so lovely. I don't want to ring this bell.

I look around, trying to figure out how to stall or back out entirely. From the corridor I see other chemo patients, rooms full of them. And then I realize something: They don't know their true prognoses any more than I do. They would *like* to hear that a man has just finished chemo, and they *want* to share in the glee. These people need to hear the bell, as hope is what we all want more than anything. Hope is the gun loaded for bear, the shot of steroids, and the hallucinogenic given to Viking raiders prior to the invasion (they got to bring home all the best-looking women, after all).

Hope is needed, so hope is given.

I ring the bell lightly. *Ding.*

"No! Ring it hard!"

She's right. I grab the chain and ring the crap out of it. *Ding, ding, ding, ding!* Finished! Made it to the other side! *Ding, ding, ding!*

A patient peeks up from his La-Z-Boy and smiles. "Last one?"

He reflects my glee and it spreads to everyone within earshot. It is an act I've performed, but it's good enough, and so everyone grins at me and each other, yelling congratulations, nodding their heads, and wondering about my hair.

This place works, their looks say, and their guns are reloaded. Wives pat husbands on their scorched, scarred, and entubed arms, for the bell has been rung and we can beat this thing.

I smile and wave weakly, feeling like a liar. Someday I'll be back.

Smokin'

Journal entry:

Happy chemo day! Last night I was quite tired at bedtime and went to sleep quickly. First I wanted to be a bit romantic with Jenelle. I suppose it grossed her out that I was chemo boy at that moment, and so my intentions went nowhere. I went through a few mental gyrations over that one, then tried to put myself in her shoes. What if she had cancer and went through chemo yesterday? Would love be on my mind? Probably, but that's me for you.

* * *

The parking spots reserved for glow-in-the-dark patients with yellow passes are full, so I park out amongst the ambulatory rabble. As I walk past the cars on Radiation Row, I see a man in the driver's seat of a Honda. Getting closer I see it's Farmer Ted waiting for his wife to finish her radiation therapy. He's smoking a cigarette.

This reminds me of when my father-in-law Jim was dying of lung cancer. He had tuberculosis as a youngster. Then he went on to smoke as an adult like all proper Irishmen. As it turns out, having tuberculosis and smoking later on in life is a good way to get small-cell lung cancer. Toward the end, a home-hospice nurse stayed with him full-time. She watched him become steadily weaker and helped him turn over to avoid sores. She cleaned his bed pan and changed out his oxygen bottle when need be. In the kitchen I asked her what it was like to work among so many dying people. She said it was tough, but that it felt good to give terminally ill cancer patients comfort. Two days before Jim died, I was leaving the house and saw her out in the driveway, smoking a cigarette. There's human nature in a nutshell.

This Mass Feels Good

After my Beast session (twenty radiations finished), I meet with Dr. The Man and Dr. Fi. I raise my arm and Dr. The Man probes for Lumpy.

"This mass feels good," he says.

Ah, I think, *that's some fine-feeling cancer*. He gives one more good jab.

"Scar tissue," he says, and removes his finger from my armpit. Then he gets a look on his face as if he just remembered something. He reaches back up and probes some more. "Didn't the surgeon remove the whole mass?" he says.

"What do you mean? No."

"No?"

"No, Doctor Young removed enough for a sample and left the rest. He said it was a tangled mess, nerves and such, all mixed in there."

The look on the face of Dr. The Man says this is all news to him. He scribbles a few notes, but does not comment further.

Dr. The Man's phone buzzes and he has to rush off to a meeting, but on his way out, he assigns a new CT scan with contrast.

I stare at the empty doorway. "Dr. Fi, what's the CT scan for?"

"This will enable us to determine just how many more radiations to apply. You are rapidly approaching the number of applications where you can begin to have harmful side effects."

"More harmful than I already have?"

"Yes," she says. "Surrounding tissue can become damaged."

This is news to me, and it's not good.

"When can you make it in for this scan?" she asks.

"How about right now?"

February 7

Journal entry:

I feel extra fuzzy this morning as though the chemo poisons are really kicking in. I seem to be able to think and write, but who knows how I'll feel about this when I read it later on?

This morning my left pinkie felt a bit numb. I don't know if I slept on it wrong or if I'm already experiencing inflammations. Oh, brother.

Jenelle comes with me to my next Dr. X appointment, which makes me happy. I explain that Dr. The Man and Dr. Fi want a CT scan to check progress. Dr. X's reply, in short, is that she will not do squat until the CT scan results are in. I discuss an Internet article I found about HPV leading to oral cancer, leading to spitting out metastases from an undetected lesion. Dr. X listens, but discounts that theory due to the lack of affected lymph nodes just downstream of the neck. However, by the time my CT scan appointment rolls around, they have me scheduled for a neck scan as well as the left axilla, so I guess I got to her and she is being extra cautious. Good!

Jenelle drives me to the hospital-side CT scan machine. I have to use that one because of scheduling conflicts with the cancer-center CT machine. We check in like mere mortals, but once the girls at the desk hear me say that I have been referred by Dr. The Man—*boom!* First-class treatment and immediate service.

A young guy and a very Texan white woman are working the CT machine today. They have me lie on the gurney the wrong way at first. I point this out.

The guy says, "Whichever way you want."

"No," I say, "it's not a matter of which way I want—it's a matter of what works properly. The previous two scans I've had were done in the opposite orientation."

This argument grows more lively, and I finally end up turned around in the original direction. After all that, I have to wonder if the guy was right and maybe it doesn't really matter.

My distress evaporates as I feel the warm caress of iodine upon my testicles.

Cars

Jenelle and I leave the CT scan and I am ecstatic! Not because of iodine floating around my naughty bits, but because The Penguin is ready—it's time to pick her up. WOO HOO! She's like brand new, including a full set of tires that I added to the tab.

Jenelle returns to work and I sneak The Penguin to the mall to meet the owner of a '95 Vette I found on Craig's List. I drive the Vette around, and it performs precisely as it should for a car that's logged 166K miles—that is, rode hard and put up wet. I like it right off the bat—it's a good-looking car. Still, it needs lots of work. What am I doing looking at a '95 Vette? Well, my Little Blue money minus the cancer bills equals one beater '95 Vette.

In the early '90s I had a '69 Malibu convertible with a 350 and factory air that actually blew cold—I'd fixed the a/c because Houston without it is a hell fest of pain, and with air conditioning, slightly less so.

I owned that car for years—it was my daily driver. It had a white interior and I put new white vinyl on the working power top. Other than a hideous paint job and the fact that she belched vast clouds of smoke whenever I started her up, she was a sweet ride.

Unfortunately for all involved, Jenelle's dashing coworker happened to own a white '89 Corvette, and he was selling it. She seemed to believe that I ought to be the owner of a nice white Corvette instead of a beater Malibu.

"No way. I'm not a Corvette guy! No gold chains, no chest hair, none of that. You're not even blonde!"

Well, she had the guy over for dinner with his girlfriend who was not blonde, and he let me drive her (the Vette, I mean). She had a six-speed manual tranny and a stout clutch, and that tranny made musical gear whine, just like a proper muscle-car. All of a sudden I was a Corvette guy; I sold the Malibu.

That Vette was, bar none, the most pain-in-the-ass car I ever owned. I spent vast amounts of time and money keeping that bitch running, and she was exceedingly difficult to work on, apparently being the demonic spawn of a Rubik's cube and a high-maintenance debutante. Just replacing spark plugs turned into a massive effort when a thread in the least accessible cylinder stripped on the way out. Oh, the sweat, the cursing, the surgery in situ! I had to pop in a helicoil just to get back on the road—and don't get me started on the heater core.

So I enter cancer treatment and suddenly crave a used Corvette. I don't just crave it, I *have* to have it! This is to be the make-up Vette—the one that makes up for all the shortcomings of the first one and magically fixes life's troubles. So what if it's derelict, with cracked gray leather seats and a very oily engine compartment, not to mention a/c that's shot. It has a lot of character; quite frankly it fits my self-image.

"Come on," I say, "how much will you take for it?"

"I have $6300 in it. I'll take $6300."

"Done." David, you master negotiator! This is proof that whatever portion of my brain which previously filtered out foolish, impulsive acts (admittedly, a weak portion of my brain in the best of times) has been pulverized by chemo and radiation.

The Vette owner pulls out his cell and arranges for a buddy to follow him while he delivers it to our house. *Well, that's nice,* I think. I give him the address and directions, thinking he'll bring it by in a day or so.

I drive straight to the bank and return home with a pile of hundred-dollar bills. The Vette and a pickup truck are already parked in front or our house, the owner standing in the driveway.

"Wow!" I say. "That was quick!"

"You brought cash?"

I look the car over one last time. *Damn, this car is pretty.* The pickup driver keeps the engine running and does not get out. While I climb around, the Vette owner fidgets and looks back toward the pickup, but when I produce the money he finally relaxes. He hands me the keys and signs the title over. I turn to admire my new toy.

"You guys want a drink or something?" I ask.

I hear the pickup's door close and by the time I turn around they are driving away. *Weird dude,* I think. *Hey, now I'm a Vette owner!*

Jenelle comes home from work and is, well, surprised to see a blue Corvette in the driveway. A heated marital debate ensues. Jenelle is angry and cannot understand why I would do such a thing. I am angry that she wouldn't want me to do such a thing. Stalemate: this discussion is going nowhere. So I play the death card: "You would deny me the last car I might ever buy?"

What a self-centered asshole I am, but I do not renege.

Doc Skin

Finally Doc Skin calls to discuss my case. He has talked over my slides with various pathologists, as well as with one of his golfing buddies at the Mayo Clinic. Long story short, he continues to be fascinated by the freakish rarity of my case. In fact, the less he is able to solve, the greater his interest appears to be. He wants to parade me in front of a bunch of cancer docs at the VA Hospital on Thursday during "Grand Rounds." I am to be the case *du jour.*

After I hang up, Jenelle asks the same question that popped into my head: Why do I need to be there in person? I suppose it's to humanize the theory and give doctors a first-hand look at me. Some big wheels from the tumor business will be there, and I will be showing off my unusual cancer.

I feel somewhat depressed, though, as Dr. Skin is wont to throw around expressions like, "We want to find the source so that you're still around," and "We don't want you to die," etc. I suppose I need to appreciate my significance to the cancer industry, but I have my own reasons to live. Like, I've got a Vette to restore!

* * *

I have felt lousy and good, from one hour to the next, over the past week since my final chemo. The side effects are not instant, they come with time, and this round is not without its own sickly charm. The fatigue is worse, and the fuzziness is worse as well.

I feel like I have not worked out in forever, even though I put in a solid workout just last Friday. I have been balancing the need for rest with my need for fitness. Rest wins for now, mostly because I have little energy and less strength.

I've had 23 radiations thus far, and will try to speak to Dr. Fi after radiation 24 tomorrow, regarding my CT scan results. I want to understand where I am and what Lumpy now looks like. I picture a cartoon raisin, flaccid and dying, covered in rad rash and looking remorseful for putting me through all this. But what if he looks like a tan Arnold Schwarze-raisin, grinning maniacally with perfect teeth?

Speaking of animated foods, Jenelle wants me to be a couch potato, but I want to be active even when I can't, so I find myself resenting her. I try to see things from her perspective—I mean, she lost her dad to cancer. And I am probably overdoing it by normal cancer standards. Jenelle loves me and wants me to stay alive, but our ideas of what is best for me do not match so we argue about it, which is yet another stressful thing about cancer.

Bonehead Goes Down

This morning is crisp and clear and I enjoy a brisk walk to the bus stop with Kaily for exercise.

All is right with the world until I go to wake up Bonehead, and she won't move. She is not comatose or asleep, but only stares at me and can't stand up. Oh, shit. Now what? If Bonehead croaks, I don't know if Kaily will be able to take it. She is still recovering from the fact that her old man has The Big C, and now her cherished pet cannot move. Dog cancer, I think. Bonehead has somehow caught cancer from me, poisoned by a mutant, contagious strain of Lumpy cells. What crap timing. I mean, can we get a break here? Jenelle offers to take Bonehead to the vet.

Sick pets aside, I snap back into a good mood because I'm going to drive my new toy to work; short attention spans have their advantages. The Vette fires right up and her exhaust note sings a happy song. Oh, yeah! When I back out I see a black oil spot the size of a grapefruit on the driveway.

On the freeway I rip right up to the speed limit. Woo-hoo! Fun! I can't help but notice that the steering wheel vibrates madly, as though the front tires were balanced by a five-year-old using bricks for weights. I make a note to check that later.

I experience a pleasant morning at the office. At the gym I do a mild workout at lunchtime. I eat a nice sandwich. I get a call from Dr. Skin's nurse as I eat a half banana. She wants to fax me directions to the VA hospital.

"Can't you just email them to me?"

"I don't have access to email."

"Oh, I'm sorry, I thought it was 2008. Can you just give me directions?"

"If I mail them to you, you won't get them in time."

"No, just read them to me over the phone." This throws her off, but I manage to coax her through it.

I am to show up on Valentine's Day at 8:00 with fifty other cancer-heads and wait for my turn. Ostensibly, I'll go up on stage and cough, or do my underwear-model pose, or juggle jugs of Berry Delicious CT scan contrast, then get sent on my way. At least that's how it sounds from Dr. Skin's vague description of the program. Even without the juggling it should be entertaining and helpful. I hope.

* * *

I arrive at the waiting room for The Beast with plenty of time to spare before zap 24. Jenelle phones before I get called back to have my face bolted down. She has Googled "trichoblastic carcinoma," a phrase that Dr. Skin dropped during his scary phone call last night (his favorite pathologist had said my lymph node biopsy slides looked trichoblastic to him). Anyhow, the trichoblastic variation of squamous cells, much like the basaloid version, can form "distant metastases." I intend to print out the article and hand it to Dr. Skin during the Grand Rounds. This prompts me to call and ask Dr. Skin's nurse for his cell phone number, just in case I run late or need to get hold of him.

She acts like I just asked for naked pictures of his wife. "That information is not given out!" she barks. Well, then!

* * *

I lie on the slab and let them bolt my head down. The iris of The Beast goes through its adjustments and gyrations, and again I feel a presence like spirits or ghosts while zoning in and out of reality. What is reality, really? I need to write that one down....

Before I chuck the gown, I find a nurse and ask to see Dr. Fi. But first, I mistakenly ask for Dr. X—I also call Kaily "Carina" a lot lately—and the nurse is confused. Then I'm also confused until figuring out my mistake. The nurse has me change clothes while she checks on Dr. Fi's availability. I see Ken in the changing room; he says he's doing well. I tell him that I am doing well too, and then I wonder if we really are.

Dr. Fi agrees to see me. She has my CT results (tabular only—no films yet), and says they show "appropriate progress." She also tells me that we have managed to avoid shrinking non-affected lymph nodes in the area. I like the sound of that. She says she will review the films, then probably "cone down," concentrating the radiation on Lumpy's epicenter (right at his nuts, I hope) for the last few treatments. She'll be working on that problem today. This makes me happy. The raisin is flaccid!

I go home and find Bonehead up and about. I'd already forgotten about her inability to rise. Jenelle tells me that Bonehead's problem is merely arthritis.

"Not cancer?" I say.

"Not cancer."

Bonehead now has a big bottle of pills that we keep by the back door. I go out and sit on the patio and pet her while looking up into the sky.

"Getting old is hell," I muse, repeating what my grandfather used to say. I look down at her sappy dog grin and realize that she doesn't give a shit about getting old—she is happy just being here, having her head stroked, living in the moment. "You stupid bonehead," I say. "You're the wisest one of all of us."

VA on V-Day

Driving through the med center is like driving through oil money; it is Dubai in Houston, the eighth wonder of the financial world. New buildings grow and spread, unstoppable, like the cancer that pays for them. I am surrounded by inspired architecture—tall spires, colossal parking garages, glass-enclosed, air-conditioned pedestrian bridges over the roadway. Business is good and the boom will never end.

Continuing forth, off in the distance I see the massive brick edifice that is the VA center. It is separated from the main medical center by the size of its parking lot, the plainness of its architecture, and the source of its funding. I drive around for quite a while, trying to figure out where to store the Penguin. I finally find an open spot, several hundred yards from the building.

I remember that it's Valentine's Day. I planned ahead and bought cards several days ago because I know how busy I am with work and medical appointments. But due to cancer-treatment brain damage, I can't remember where I put them; I looked everywhere for them last night. I'll have to go buy some more.

The day is clear and cool; clouds wisp across the sky, golden in the sunrise. I ponder the Grand Rounds. Dr. Skin will presumably describe my case and I am guessing that people will gawk, expecting someone who looks cancerous, while I show off Lumpy. It's Bring Your Tumor to Work Day! I am telling myself to maintain low expectations, or perhaps have none, just let a new experience unfold before me.

Afterward, I will have radiation at 4:00 PM—it's usually 4:45, but I'm supposed to show up early to get a body mold made that will allow me to lie there in a new underwear model position while they zap me with a more concentrated beam, right at the cancer site. As of yesterday, I've had 25 radiations.

I think about the times when I was strapped down by the head on the radiation table, and wonder how I ever fell asleep in that position. This happened fairly often, in fact, and now strikes me as quite odd.

At 8:00 I enter the VA. This hospital is freaking huge, filled to the brim with the uncelebrated side of war: disabled veterans. There are lots of wheelchairs, walkers and canes, guys with limps and missing parts, and long lines everywhere—especially wherever cancer patients have to go, such as the lab for blood work. It is sad.

Mostly I see Vietnam-era vets, but there are some old guys from WWII and Korea still kicking, and various survivors of Iraq and Afghanistan—dudes who look as young as Carina.

Grand Rounds

At 8:20 I'm escorted to my own exam room and told to wait with my shirt off. For a while, nothing happens other than me shivering, but then comes the stampede. Several dozen interns, doctors, pharmaceutical reps, and their cousins, in-laws and wives flood through and look me over. I'm an interesting specimen! About half of them probe my underarm, often without asking permission. They feel for Lumpy but ignore his host. I wonder if the World's Shortest Man feels this way, or maybe the Bearded Lady.

I am not supposed to tell the gawkers and probers anything about my case—they are supposed to figure it out—but I don't learn this until after a half dozen or so onlookers have felt up Lumpy.

Dr. Skin arrives in my exam room; he is all excited by the interest in my case. I give him the trichoblastic carcinoma article that Jenelle found. At first he dismisses it out of hand (*Hey, hey, don't be solving this shit—it's the only joy I have!*), but then he seems to consider it. He leaves and brings in a couple of seasoned professionals who also probe my underarm without asking first. Their age makes me feel happy.

The probers suddenly dry up as quickly as they came. I am instructed by a nurse to put my shirt on and leave. What, no on-the-spot cure? I feel cheap and used, probed and dumped.

I walk around the ground floor a bit more, feeling a greater empathy for the poor damaged bodies and patient souls in the endless lines.

My grandfather had a saying: "Everyone should own a convertible once in their life. Pretty much cures them of it." I have a corollary: "Everyone who finds war to be grand and stirring should spend a morning at a VA hospital. Pretty much cures them of it."

* * *

I pose for my fresh body mold. Nurse WW scootches me around into my new underwear model pose, then realigns me a few times. She and Dr. Fi paint some blue dots and an X on my chest. The mold is cast and allowed to harden. I have yet another CT scan to help them aim the new radiation pattern. This body mold is to be used for the last five zaps, during which I will not have my head bolted to a slab of steel. Where's the fun in that?

At 5:45 I stand in our den and remove my shirt to look at the dots and the X. I'm a living map for buried treasure that will surely be radioactive by the end of all this. I grab the digital camera and take a self-portrait, then wander upstairs to the computer to upload the photo. I'm horrified at what I see on the screen. *Holy crap!* I'm all skin and bones! I have sunken cheeks! When did this happen, and how come I never noticed? I can see Lumpy's scar under my left armpit—it is now flat, vaginal no more. I can also see that my left lat and pec muscles have been bitch-slapped by The Beast.

Luckily for skinny me, Jenelle and I have a big steak dinner planned in Cupid's honor.

But I am leaving out the good news: Between the body mold and now, I saw Dr. X. She said that, based on the CT scan of last Thursday, Lumpy's lease has been revoked. It is hereby null and void. Probably. In other words, my body has responded as desired to the treatment and the cancerous mass in my left axilla has shrunken down to a bit of scar tissue and some atrophied muscles. Of course there's been collateral damage to my psyche tantamount to that produced by a cluster bomb, but Lumpy is dead. Probably. We'll know for sure after my next PET scan.

So, am I deliriously happy? No. I'm fairly happy, but it is happiness tainted with disappointment. *What the hell?* you might well ask. *Where is the Champagne, you ungrateful survivor? Some Lance Armstrong you are!*

Here is the problem, and it weighs upon me heavily: My partner that I have known and loved for all these years has betrayed me. Not Jenelle, but my body. I have trusted my body and treated it well – aside from those 20,000 beers, countless tequila shots, and various assaults of junk food and sleep deprivation. And I took only a few nasty spills while showing off on skis. Yet after all that care and consideration, my body let Lumpy in.

The point being: if my body did it once, what's to stop it from doing it again? So the best cheer I can work up at the moment is a cautious optimism for the PET scan and future scans thereafter. The experts are 100% certain that Lumpy metastasized from elsewhere. Perhaps the primary cancer no longer exists, as Dr. Skin and Dr. X theorize. Perhaps it does. Who knows?

But one thing is certain: Lumpy is puny and may be gone for good, probably no longer posing a threat of further metastases. This is a big load off, but not a full load. I will take it because I have no choice.

So, will I become healthy again and resume normal life? Maybe after my last radiations (precautionary, I am assured, to make Lumpy triple-extra dead), followed by a few weeks of post-radiation recovery. What about my disappointment and lingering anxiety and other mental problems? Bah! What kind of pansy has mental problems after cancer, especially entry-level cancer?

Tsunami

The unofficial news of Lumpy's likely death spurs an interesting phenomenon. I am awakened by an urge about an hour before my alarm is supposed to go off. It is not the urge to have sex or to fly, for those urges never truly recede; it is the urge to go to the bathroom, for I am obliged to drink a lot of water. But going to the bathroom is not the interesting phenomenon, it is what happens afterward.

I have lately been calm enough to go right back to sleep after a trip to Mr. Toilet—day at a time and all that—without letting the minutiae of daily life get beyond my impenetrable shield of OPP (Other People's Problems). Oh yes, sometimes I worry about cancer, mortality, and the meaning of life, but that is understandable.

In the wee hours of this morning, however, it has sunk in that I am probably not going to die of cancer, at least not in the short term. So instead of going back to sleep, a cascade of not-going-to-die bullshit comes flooding into my head: *What about the drawings*

I need at work? Are there enough chairs in our house to seat everyone at Easter? Should I fix the Corvette a/c now or wait until it gets good and hot? I have to avoid the sun. Will I catch a cold? What day is my nadir? What's my white cell count? Is my sperm radioactive and chemically altered? I should set up a nice garage workshop. Which gym should I go to today? Can I go back to sleep now? Okay, how about now? And on and on....

My alarm goes off like a buzz-saw at 6:15; no sleep has occurred after the bathroom trip. I try to be philosophical, chalking up the thought-tsunami to pent-up crap that must be purged, but this is ridiculous. Where is the serenity I deserve after facing down death?

A Spanking

Journal entry:

I feel weak and puny right now—that began last night right after supper.

Others may look at my life and see obvious signs of why I got cancer. I do not. We all swim in our own worlds of cause and effect, not seeing the connections, but wondering why bad things happen to us.

On the other hand, is this cancer somehow a good thing? I would have never entertained that notion in my life B.C., but now things feel differently; Lumpy has shifted the tectonic plates of my soul. My view of what's important and what isn't has certainly changed; I'm more willing to let go of little things, as the Chicken Soup books advise. Is a greater happiness possible for me now? Maybe.

But there are still plenty of not-good things about getting cancer: My physical well-being is now compromised by skewed blood-cell counts. Other side-effects of radiation and chemotherapy still seem to be waging a war of attrition on my body. I have photographic proof that I am fashion-model skinny, and I did not have a lot of extra weight to give in the first place.

Fortunately the chemo is over and there are only six more

radiations, only one of which will be contributing to my rad-rash, which is itchy and dry right now, somewhat like poison ivy.

I made my skinny self do a ten-minute workout yesterday on the heavy bag (I hung it in the garage, and it felt about as heavy as I am). The workout was good and loud, as the closed garage doors formed a nice acoustic chamber. The neighbor kids playing basketball probably thought I was spanking a bag of wet cement with a canoe paddle; they always thought I was a little strange, even more so recently. The cement spanking was rigorous and may have contributed to today's weakness, thus bolstering Jenelle's argument for rest. Anyhow, here I am, up a couch without a paddle.

I got a call from Dr. Skin yesterday (or Saturday, I cannot recall which—this sort of memory lapse is the norm lately). Doc Skin, in a nutshell, said nothing definitive. But he talked for twenty minutes and threw out some nice tidbits, especially: Good prognosis. His colleagues at the Grand Rounds feel it's a stretch to think that anything other than a local cancer source, something right there in Lumpy's neighborhood, could have affected me. The phrases "long shot" and "low odds" were tossed around.

Does this make me happy? Not really. This whole freaking ordeal has been a "long shot" and there were "low odds" that I would get cancer in the first place. So I do not see why the Grand Rounds armpit probers should feel so surprised that I am bucking their trends. Anyhow, I'm supposed to provide Dr. Skin's office with a release form today so that he may acquire the report from a messy and involved sun-damage basal-cell removal from my forehead, done during a Valium-saturated operation called Mohs surgery in the year 2000. I remember Jenelle telling me that I had a patch of skin cut out about the size of a quarter, and also that I was quite happy about it, due to the drugs. The doctor pulled what was left of my forehead skin back together and sewed it up. It left a really cool scar that makes me look tough, or at least clumsy. Dr. Skin thinks that this report will hold the key to this fun and intriguing mystery— the smoking tissue, as it were.

Rad Rash

Journal entry:

I finished my last MESH FACE, face-mask radiation yesterday! WOO HOO! That was #28. As of this moment, I have 5 radiations left, and they are of the easy variety, concentrated on the cancerous region only.

I brought my radiation face mask home yesterday. It's now sitting on the kitchen counter with some sunglasses on it. Kaily says it looks like me.

Today is my blood-count nadir from the second chemo, and it feels like it. I don't feel pain or nausea, but a general lack of energy and will. Rad rash has now spread like an extreme case of poison ivy, extending from my neck to my chest and around my shoulder and upper back on the Lumpy side. It keeps me awake at night and is generally an itchy, nasty business, which I blame on Lumpy.

I also feel a swollen lymph node on the left where my back meets my lower neck. I am hoping it is swollen due to the rash, but will ask Dr. The Man during my consultation, just in case he irradiated me into yet more cancer, or Lumpy up and moved instead of dying. Fortunately this lymph node is a bit squishy, not the frozen blueberry variety.

I venture into the office for an ordinary day at the grindstone and wind up having a great breakthrough. There is a design that has been vexing me for about a week, and suddenly the answer has come to me. I love it when that happens! Clouds part and life is no longer grim or depressing. Maybe I will get through this after all.

* * *

Dr. The Man looks over my chart, and informs me that I only have three more radiations, not five, the first of which is today. Hell yes! Two less!

My session with The Beast is at 2:45. I lay down in my new body cast, sans face mask, and kick back for a proper broiling in Underwear Model Pose #2. These are not "light" radiations, mind you; there is more than one station over thirty-seconds long, maybe three stations, but I cannot remember, even right after.

There are somewhere around five stations altogether. The old setup had seven stations, I think, but I cannot remember that either.

I come away from my intense round of rays in a good mood with a short-term memory comparable to that of a dope-smoking Alzheimer's patient.

For the rest of the afternoon, I feel euphoric.

I drop Kaily off at taekwondo and return home. Jenelle is already at the house, and we talk about my treatment and apparently continuing life. Since the news is better lately, we feel liberated to use more words. I feel well enough to tinker with the driver's-side headlight on the Vette which, much like its owner, exhibits intermittent wackiness. The headlight stays open when it's supposed to close and my car looks like it's winking. I cannot figure out how to fix it, either because I'm flighty or because it's a Corvette.

I go to pick Kaily up, still feeling good. I talk to Mike, another taekwondo student, and tell him of my cancer. It turns out that he already knew, but not in accurate detail. Then, when Kaily and I are about to leave, BOOM!—my whole being crashes, feeling weak and tired beyond all reason. This seems to be the pattern. Fine, fine, fine, *crash*. And I have not exercised, therefore too-much-physical-activity is not a suspect. I figure that it is either my blood count or the newly intense radiation, or both.

Crash aside, today was still a beautiful day. Things are looking up.

The Last Zap

Nurse Wonder Woman tells me that I need no more CBCs. I'm gonna miss filling up those vials with my fine cabernet, and the women who salivate over my veins before plunging needles into my arm up to the hilt. Ahh... the good old days.

Today is my last zap, then they can stick a fork in me because I'll be done. Oh, I'll have a follow-up PET scan and other doctor visits in about a month, but today treatment officially ends.

I bring flowers and cards for the receptionist and the Women of Radiation (sounds like a Playboy cover story), plus cards for Dr. Fi and Dr. The Man. I'm giddy with anticipation. There are a few newbies in the waiting room and I can tell they are wondering just what the hell is going on here, and why I'm so happy and toting gifts. I just grin.

I don the gown and give the nurses their flowers. They seem as giddy as I am. I lay upon my La-Z-Boy body mold and smile at The Beast.

"Hurt me, cook me, call me darlin'!"

By now my rad rash is focused in a smaller region, but is red as hell and itchier than ever. Also, there are new bits of aching and tightness down my left arm, and a dark, almost bruised area under my left armpit. Basically, they are hammering the crap out of the cancer epicenter and Lumpy's dead body. I am not opposed to this.

I count: Twenty-eight seconds, fifteen seconds—these are full-strength, focused, harsh, cooking zaps. The next station is thirty or so seconds, and I begin to lose focus. I continue to count seconds on the final few stations, but cannot remember the answer or even how many stations there are.

I run in the meadow of the scene on the ceiling; the breeze blows; butterflies flit by. Fluffy clouds move overhead and take the shape of J-Lo's most famous anatomical feature. The slab jerks, The Beast's head retracts, and I am finished.

8 ACCELERATION

I back the Corvette out of Radiation Row and idle over to the freeway access road. When the traffic clears I floor the pedal. Both rear tires shriek, sending burnout smoke skyward along with my Ohio-transplant rebel yell straight out of the *Dukes of Hazzard* (Dukes of Dayton?). YEEE-HAAA!!!

The tail end of the Vette kicks left while I go right, propelled by radioactive V8 power overload. We launch, nay, *rip* screaming away from cancer, The Beast, and chemo, lurching forward onto the highway of life.   The Vette hits sixty before I have a nagging, decelerating thought: Did all that treatment really "take"? Did it do anything at all? Am I actually better—or do I have a new, superbug strain of cancer hiding out in my tissues, a mutated Lumpy who eats chemo for breakfast and laughs at mere radiation, waiting to kill me a little later when my guard is down?

No! More gas, more speed; I'll outrun this doubt.   But seriously, I do not know, and I am not allowed to have a PET scan for a month in order to avoid false positives. Hello limbo, my old friend. On the other hand: F_ _ _ cancer! I hit ninety before I have to jam on the brakes for a red light.

Zapped and Sapped

Journal entry:

Here I sit, not a cancer visit for the next 3 weeks, not even a CBC or anything! Done!

Being free of The Beast sends me into euphoria. No more succulent bags of poison; I am ready to traipse through the translucent mountain scene, to feel like I'm nineteen, strong and invincible once more.

But traipsing is not really an option, mostly because I am wrung out. Apparently the Beast's venom takes a day or two to sink in after the last treatment. My shoulder is puffy and sore, and blood counts are low, so I still couldn't go to the gym if I had the energy. The final radiation sessions, which I thought would be easy, have knocked me on my ass. I have found a new level *below* tired: zapped and sapped. And, oh yes, fuzzy. I have become intimate with the term "radiation poisoning."

I am skinnier and weaker than ever, and feel neither nineteen nor immortal. More like ninety and on borrowed time. But still there is an ember glowing deep down in my tired-ass soul. And that ember has a voice, and that voice keeps saying: *F_ _ _ cancer!* So I decide to quit lying on the couch, watching a hi-definition TV show about people surviving ordeals of nature, and see if I can survive walking out to the front porch in normal definition. I do, but feel puny and winded.

From here, surely I can make it to the mailbox. I go back inside and grab the mailbox key and go down the front path, pleased that I can still walk. I make it to the street with no physical pain, only a bit of labored breathing and a deep-seated desire to return to the couch and sleep for a few hours. The ember taunts me: *Keep going, you wimp!* I don't take that sort of abuse from any ember and make it to the mailbox on pure stubbornness. Then I make it all the way home without keeling over, so f_ _ _ cancer, and up yours, ember!

The next morning I walk Kaily a few blocks to the bus stop and then walk all the way back home. I'm a god! So what if my breathing feels like I've been jogging, and I'm a bit dizzy. But now I feel only seventy years old instead of ninety. The next morning I make the same bus stop trip and add a journey around the neighborhood, taking the long way back to the house. Now I'm only sixty-five and ready to retire.

I walk farther and faster each day, dropping decades and

feeling better. Working my muscles even in this relatively minor way seems to help purge my system of chemicals and surplus neutrons. Days pass; lungs pump less; counts creep upward. Walking really works!

I plan a visit to the gym soon, and expect to return to taekwondo after Easter. The key word here is "plan." I can plan for the future now—not very far, but more than a day or two. For example, Jenelle and I are hosting Easter this year for the whole family, and I tell my father and brother to bring their golf clubs. I make plans for the Corvette and the garage. It is refreshing to feel such hope.

Springing Forth

Time passes and I continue to feel better. I seem to have passed some flush-out milestone for Cisplatin and radiation, and judging by my energy levels, my blood counts must be back up as well. Sometimes. Evenings I still crash, and crash hard.

There is a long list of side effects from chemo and radiation, but mostly they come down to being tired—profoundly tired—a dead tiredness that settles in as pain at the base of my skull. And a general feeling of toxicity, like a low-level flu, pervades my body. A few times a week I wake up in the middle of the night obsessed with inanities and cannot go back to sleep, which makes me even more tired.

But all is not lost, for there is a simple solution: coffee. I self-medicate by downing copious quantities of java; it seems to negate the radiation flu. When it wears off, I drink some more. And some more. Pretty soon I'm keeping a caffeine buzz on all during the workday, and before you know it I've got Juan Valdez on my back: a massive caffeine addiction. I work while drinking black coffee; then exercise, finished off by espresso; then putter around the house before a glass of iced coffee with honey and soymilk. This can't be a bad thing—I mean, how toxic is coffee compared to chemo and radiation? It's like a crack addict switching to M&Ms; it's child's play. No worries, and it works! Except for the insomnia, flashes of anxiety, bursts of hyperactivity, and unannounced crashes from whence I groggily awake with my head on my desk.

I push hard and suffer accordingly. My cancer shoulder aches as I crash and re- caffeinate in regular cycles, tempting system-wide exhaustion from trying to exercise, work, and live normally without enough sleep. I should listen to Jenelle, but the more she wants me to rest the more I rebel. What the hell has gotten into me? I feel a bit crazy, but cannot put my finger on it, and sometimes wonder if I've imagined the whole thing: Life, that is.

On the Ides of March, Dr. X sees me and finally assigns the PET scan that will offer official proof of whether all this treatment actually worked or not. But I have to wait for that scan until April 11, then wait even longer for results.

"It's okay to exercise," she says.

"Good," I say, "because I'm already doing that."

"Your lymph nodes feel normal," she says. "And the left axilla is healing as expected."

The world moves on and time keeps passing, and I continue to regain strength and *joie de vivre*. Springtime comes and with it green grass, little yellow flowers, optimism and hope, and lots of rain. I exercise and live and work and drink coffee.

One particularly lovely spring morning, I decide to enhance the joy of life by going for a drive in the Corvette. Alas, it won't start. I hook up the charger but find that the battery is fully charged. I turn the key and the dash lights come on as though everything is fine. Still, the starter won't turn. Enthusiasm ebbs as I stare at the byzantine engine compartment before closing the hood. *Holy crap, how the hell am I going to figure this out?*

I find a Corvette forum online and discover that my car has a magical ignition key with a built-in electronic chip, which prevents theft by valets who would make copies of my key while I'm eating dinner. Their copies would have no chip, of course. *Ha, ha,* we owners of '90s GM cars think, *we are a little too clever for you!* However, this ingenious system for thwarting criminals has one problem: eventually the chip reader in the ignition switch wears out, and the engine won't start for the owner. Further research will be required to find out how I can steal my own car. I drive the Penguin in the meantime.

The calendar rolls over to April, and I make my post-treatment debut at taekwondo class. Things go well in the *dojang*. I am pleased to be able to attend class without injuring anything. People treat me fairly normally, so I guess Master Steel Curtain hasn't told *everybody*. I survive the pushups and ab work and drills with less difficulty than anticipated, mostly because I have low expectations. All that gym training, plus Jenelle-ordered rest over Easter weekend, has worked in my favor. Kaily and I get home after 9:00 and the two-headed shower feels exceptionally luxurious. I follow this with a big meal and sleep like a baby.

* * *

I find that doing internet research is much more enjoyable when it does not involve Googling my own prognosis. I discover an article that describes how to steal my own Corvette: snip a small wire under the dash and twist in a dollar's worth of Radio Shack resistors, thus bypassing the magical chip reader entirely. It works! The key now starts the car! I post my success online. Purists reply that I must stop this insanity and buy a new chip-reading ignition switch for several hundred dollars. This Radio Shack method, they say, invites certain theft, as well as rendering my Vette "non-factory-original" by using cobbled-together parts. "Why don't you just duct tape a giant spoiler on the back?" one purist laments. "Then bolt a giant set of steer horns onto the hood." I decide to live with the risk and the stigma.

I drive the Vette to work the next day, starting the engine at will and feeling quite smug. On the way home I stop for groceries. When I attempt to leave the store the shifter won't work properly and I cannot get the Vette into reverse. I settle for neutral, leave the car running, and push it out of the parking spot. I manage to yank the shifter into "Drive" with an absurd amount of force before I feel the mechanism pop. Now the shifter moves with ease, so much that it won't settle into any other gear. *What now?* Fortunately the transmission is permanently stuck in drive and I'm pointed in the correct direction. I make it home and have to shut the car off still in gear, and can't even get my formerly magical key out. There is no time to sort through it, though. I need to make more time.

What about cancer? Just say no! I do not want to think of

cancer while I wait for my PET scan! Only work and exercise and coffee, my man cave and my Vette. I plunge headlong into distraction with as much intensity as I've applied to my fight with Lumpy.

A week passes with many of my off hours spent in the garage. I've installed floor cabinets and hung wall cabinets, and added a shorty workbench; the place is looking good. I've torn into the Vette as well, tracing its inability to shift to an inexpensive cable.

When my new shift cable arrives via UPS, I climb under the Vette to install it. Oh yes, piece of cake! The old cable is held to the transmission with a few clips and bolts. I love working on my old Corvette! So simple!

But that is only one end of the cable. While still under the car, I find that the other end snakes into the passenger compartment, and is attached from that side with three screws; I can see their pointy little ends poking down from above. *That looks easy enough,* I think.

I climb into the driver's seat and have no idea how to find the three screws. I pull off a trim piece beside the shifter. Still no screws. I go to pull off another trim piece and find that it won't come off without removing yet another piece just above the steering wheel, but that won't come off without pulling off an oddly shaped piece just above the gauges. I'm going in the wrong direction! I remove these pieces and more, and still can't see the screws.

This goes on and on with layers upon layers of trim pieces and plastic bits. I work for over an hour and still haven't uncovered the shift-cable screws, but have now removed the following: a fair amount of the dash, both seats, most of the console and two large pieces of carpet that go on either side of the console. I have an old olive jar halfway full of trim screws.   I discover that the seat track on the driver's side needs to be repaired.

I stare at the mess and my gut reaction is despair. I try to flip that around and take the opposite view. This car is a symbol of *optimism*. Taking on a long-term project like this means I hope to be alive to finish it. It occurs to me that this car is also a symbol of myself, my body, my life. I needed somebody to work on me, and probably still do. If I were this far taken apart, I'd like to have new carpet and seat covers when I was put back together. I decide to order some online. Time to go relax for the night.

After work the next day I march straight out to the symbol of optimism and continue repairing myself. After another half hour and several more trim bits and pieces, I still cannot see the three shift-cable screws. I suspect that they are under the radio. Now how do I get that out? Careful study is required and various tools are scrounged from the dusty back corners of my toolbox.

When the radio is out, I can finally see the three bolts. But they are under a piece of dash structure that renders them inaccessible to tools. The wind deserts my sails as it dawns on me that I'll have this car dismantled to the molecular level by the time I gain access to these damned screws. I decide that I don't really love working on my old Corvette; somehow I've managed to dismantle my optimism.

There is but one solution: coffee! I plop down with a cup of Joe on the bare floor of my fun toy, staring at the remaining structure above the bolts, then the pile of console, shifter, and trim pieces and loose carpet, and the full jar of screws. I hear a heavy sigh from my own chest. But when all appears lost, the ember kicks in: *You're gonna let this car beat you?*

No! I climb back out and return with a drill sporting a large bit. *Corvette purists be damned!* Soon the shift-cable screws are accessible via fresh holes, and in another minute and a half I have the old cable pulled out. Victory! Well...half a victory. I still have to put this mess back together.

* * *

Some days are better than others, and most seem overly stuffed with tasks: work at Firm D; work on the garage; write; journal; exercise. Where is the free time earned by my victorious dance with death? My journals from these weeks reveal my affair with fatigue:

tired as hell right now, but a little less fuzzy today...
woke up in the middle of the night and thought...
fuzzy-headed, fell asleep in front of the TV...
a little less extra tired right now...
tired as hell, no time...

While I await the new Corvette carpet and seat covers, my pendulum swings the other way: I decide to avoid distractions for a while and instead live in the moment. I find shapes in clouds and feel the breeze on a grassy hill at dusk. Thoughts of cancer creep back in and I ponder Lumpy's short life and my own mortality, especially as my PET scan approaches. I'll be obliged to patiently await results, and in the meantime try to go about in blissful ignorance. I watch sunrises. By now I cannot be bothered to fret over the mundane flotsam and jetsam of daily life—only over my PET scan. I fret over that a lot.

April 11

This PET scan goes the same as the first—I am complimented on my veins, I endure the injection of radioactive goo, I wait one hour in the waiting chamber, I watch the Phillip's head screws as I jut in and out of the scan machine. Been there, done that.   The scan is easy now; old hat. Waiting for results is when the furies emerge. Or try to.

In order to survive and not go insane with anxiety, I find myself letting things go and relaxing more in the face of situations that used to stress me out. Trying to be normal and busy takes energy, but this new let-it-be philosophy helps. I find myself enjoying the days—all of them. Sure, anxiety still overcomes me at times. But those times are individual battles; I'm still winning the war.

Lance Theory

Suddenly my Livestrong bracelet breaks. I am shocked and don't know how to react. It just lies there on the floor, a broken strap instead of a bracelet. Is my life over?

Maybe not – maybe my life has just begun. As suddenly as my bracelet broke, I realize that I don't want to replace it. I could use Jenelle's or ask for another one, but I don't want to; I no longer want to be reminded of what it's about. Treatment has ended and I no longer want to immerse myself in cancer lore. I don't want to forget it all forever, but I do want to forget for a while. I want to achieve normalcy, whatever that is. (I'll keep the mask, though.)

I continue to drink coffee. Not a lot of coffee, but *absurd quantities* of coffee, to fight the fatigue and feign normalcy. Life goes on, and I live strongly without a bracelet, as long as there's enough caffeine.

I believe that exercise will save me, as it helped save Lance. That's why throughout this ordeal I exercised like crazy, unless I was knocked on my ass by low counts or treatment after-effects. I was glad to be able to walk around the neighborhood after the hard-core radiation finale, winded and wimpy.

Now I'm back at the gym. At first it was a couple of days a week with puny amounts of weight befitting a pitiful cancer patient, but I quickly ramped up to many days weekly working out madly. I *am* a madman; I want to purge all memories of the cancer and the treatment. I believe so much that exercise will save me that I fight with Jenelle if she so much as hints that I should take it easy. *F_ _ _ that*, I think, and *f_ _ _ cancer!*

I am quite possibly delusional. I was in the best shape of my life when I was diagnosed; the same goes for Lance. Therefore my belief that exercise will prevent cancer is loopy twice over. But I believe anyhow. I believe that exercise kept my cancer from being worse than it was. If cancer is a voracious consumer of glucose, then I will make my muscles even greater consumers of glucose. I want my muscles to burn glucose like Hummers burn oil.

My desire, nay, my *obsession* to kill cancer—to use up all the glucose and do whatever else is required to stay alive—gives me insight into Lance Armstrong's ability to win the Tour de France. I call it my Lance Theory. The maddening thought that my body has been violated by cancer—a cellular form of rape—plus the weird transformations brought about by chemotherapy and radiation have turned me into an exercise monster, a Frankenstein on a self-healing rampage. The French press accused Mr. Armstrong of various doping strategies. I know that dope was not only unnecessary, but wouldn't have done the job anyway. The man's secret was cancer.

Results

On the evening before my PET scan results, I eat the best lasagna I've ever had with Carina at an Italian restaurant in Rice Village, and it makes me happy. Carina gives me a tour of KTRU Rice Radio where she is a DJ, and that makes me happy too. When we show up there is a guy in the DJ chair doing his gig, a blues show. It is genuinely cool, this radio station—graffiti on the walls, endless shelves of vinyl, and tons of CDs. It exceeds my expectations of college radio. I enjoy seeing it the same way I now enjoy almost anything besides cancer and the memories of treatment. I love life and my newfound ability to soak up all that I can.

Then I remember that it is one day until my PET scan results. I try to cling to the idea of no expectations. I want this day to end on the same happy note I picked up at the station. I drive home and glance in on the Corvette. It is now back together and ready to drive, with new carpeting and seat covers. All is well; my Optimism has been remodeled. Right before bedtime I notice that Dr. Otherdermo's office girl has left a cell-phone message.

"Uhm, Mr. Baskwinn? Dr. Otherdermo looked at your blood test results? He needs to see you in person? To discuss them?"

Aside from the girl butchering my last name and embracing the trend of making all statements into questions, I find this phone call unnerving because blood test results that require a personal visit cannot be happy blood test results. This message cuts short the lingering happy note, and makes me wish I were at the gym exercising. Or out drinking.

* * *

My appointment to see Dr. X for post-treatment PET scan results finally arrives. It is Friday morning. I wait by myself on crinkly white paper atop the Ritter 204 exam table, and try not to worry about whether I should be worried. I keep waiting. I wish that Jenelle were here, but she's at work. I try to understand why she picked work over supporting me, and I decide that it is a mitigation strategy. If I croak, she'll need a solid career to pay for the giant house. This is not a comforting line of thought, so I must be worrying. Then again, maybe she just fears the results too much to be here. Now I'm definitely worrying.

The door opens and Dr. X comes in still reading my report. She glances up.

"All clear," she says, right off the bat.

I exhale a big one. She keeps reading.

"Oh," she exclaims, "wait!" I find myself unable to inhale as she peers at the page in front of her. "Well, yes," she says offhandedly, leafing through more pages, "your left axilla is all clear, cancer's gone, but there's this other little something."

WTF!?

There is another pause while she continues reading. My body says, *Hey man! How about if we inhale?* So I do, which enables me to speak: "What other little something?"

"The PET scan shows some activity on your left vocal cord," she says with a frown before finally looking up. "Might just be allergies, though."

My mind leaps to Warp Factor 7, which all Trekkies know means seven times the speed of light.   *Left vocal cord = throat = squamous cells*, which means that we have just found Lumpy's father! I sit in stunned silence.

"You don't seem very happy about your left axilla," Dr. X observes.

"Uhm, yes, ecstatic. It's just that, well, should I not be panicking about throat cancer?"

"Oh, no," she says, "like I said, it could be nothing. It's best not to worry until you know for sure. It's probably nothing."

In fact it's so "probably nothing" that Dr. X calls Dr. Uvula to work me in for an immediate throat scoping. I check out and wander into the parking lot. Where am I? Oh yeah, cancer center. Where the hell did I park and which car did I drive?

So now I might have cancer in my throat.   But I might not. How does this make me feel? Well, what I wanted to hear was "all clear" without caveats or exceptions. Instead I have *activity* on my left vocal cord—what is that about? Lumpy's dad is dancing? Humping? What *kind* of activity? I find that I've driven the Corvette, because there it is parked, and I manage to unlock it and sit on the driver's side. I alternate between staring blankly at my phone and peering blankly through the windshield before calling Jenelle at work to tell her the news.

"I don't know where I'll find strength for this," I confess. I'm crying a bit.

"No, you'll be fine. It's good news about your axilla. You're fine. That's good! It's probably nothing." She stops talking; I hear sniffles.

I start the Corvette and remember wrecking the Penguin on the pole. Drivin' the car? *Drivin' the car.* I stop at a STOP sign; good idea. If Dr. Uvula does, indeed, find cancer on my left vocal cord, it will at least jibe with the cancer in my left axilla, and provide a more convincing source for same than skin cancer. Drivin' the car? *Tryin'.* The downside would be another, probably more heinous round of chemo and radiation. Drivin' the car? *Feelin' nauseous.*

Odds are that the little something will be allergies, but I have beaten odds the wrong way before—so I am gun-shy and skeptical about just how *fine* I am.

It is only 10:15 AM when I arrive at the practice of Dr. Uvula. At this point I have no choice but to go through the motions and see what happens. Walking up the stairs, I suddenly remember the message from Dr. Otherdermo's office about needing to see him in person regarding blood-test results. With all of the throat news I'd forgotten and didn't even bring it up with Dr. X. Now it's WTF all over again. My legs feel heavy. Will this shit never end?

I enter the waiting room where Fox News blares—no, I guess this shit will never end. I'm wishing for a shotgun when I get called back to the exam room.

Dr. U's nurse brings in a laptop. "What are you here for?"

"I might have cancer in my throat," I say, "or I may be fine, and it's nothing." She types this in.

"Are you on any medication?"

"No."

She types that in, too, but with lots of keystrokes. Maybe she's emailing somebody. "You're supposed to get scoped?"

"Yes."

She types that in, then leaves and then comes back and squirts the vile hell goo into both nostrils. The squirt device sounds like an airbrush. The goo runs out both nostrils and fills the single Kleenex she has provided me with. She leaves again and I wait.

Dr. Uvula enters and I stand to shake his hand, but have to throw away the Kleenex first.

"How are you doing?" he says, and seems to actually care.

"I was hoping you'd tell me." I tell him the story of the PET scan and what Dr. X has said about it, and the "activity" in my throat.

Doc U fires up the little black snake and shoves it into my right nostril several inches, then several more for good measure. I feel it clanging around in the tonsil region. I try not to look at my throat, but there it is, on TV in pink. He has me squeeze my nostrils and sing "EEEE!" He twists the snake and snaps a couple of pictures.

"Hmm..." he murmurs, sliding the snake back up and out. "You're all clear," he says calmly. "False alarm."

I do not feel like asking him if he's sure, and instead feel like buying him a twenty-five-year-old single-malt Scotch. As I leave I feel the heaviness fall away. I call Jenelle and we both scream and laugh into our phones. Then I remember.

"One more thing," I tell her. "Now I just have to go to Dr. Otherdermo and find out why he wants to discuss my blood in person." I hear the other end go silent. "Sorry," I say. "Not trying to be a downer, just factual."

"When's your appointment?"

"Oh, I get to wait until Monday for that one."

* * *

Over the weekend, I wait and wonder over all the good news, bad news, changing news, and news yet to come. When Monday arrives, I can be found sitting in Dr. Otherdermo's waiting room reading the latest *Texas Monthly* I can find, seventeen months old, while videos play in an endless loop above me. The first video is of two teenagers with bad acne, and one old man with various old-man skin blotches. They all become happy by visiting their friendly dermatologist. The next video is of an old lady being zapped by lasers, and then looking happy and years younger. Instead of looking seventy-three, now she looks only sixty-nine.

I get called back to an exam room to wait some more. I don't feel like playing with the electric exam table, so I just lay back and stare at the ceiling. *What now?* I wonder. After twenty more minutes spent pointlessly playing with the old cell phone, Dr. Otherdermo comes in holding my file. We exchange greetings.

"Well?" I say.

"Well what?" he says, looking through my paperwork.

"What blood results do you need to see me about?"

He stops looking through the paperwork and stares at me a moment. "What are you talking about?"

"Your receptionist said you have to go over some blood-test results in person, so I know they must be bad. Do I have melanoma?"

"I don't know what she meant by that," he replies. "I only need to remove a bit more skin from the base of your neck. The pathology showed some more sun damage, and I want to make sure I get it all."

I have to wait a moment to absorb this. "There are no bad blood-test results?"

"Nope," he answers, "no bad blood-test results."

"What? Holy crap, Doc! Your phone girl left me a message saying you had to go over blood test results in person! She scared the shit out of me!"

We talk it over and he apologizes and says he'll make sure it doesn't happen again. I calm down.

"Sorry for losing my temper, Doc."

He nods. "I would say it's no skin off my back," he smiles, "but I'm about to take some off yours and you might not think that's funny." No shit.

He has me remove my shirt and shoots Lidocaine near the base of my neck. The needle stings, but I am so used to needles by now that I barely notice. He scrapes, patches me up, then sends me on my way.

Finally, on the drive home, I relax. No cancer. *No cancer.* NO CANCER! For now, at least. But that bastard Lumpy still has me spooked. F-ing Lumpy! F_ _ _ cancer!

May 1

May Day! I feel unwell, as if I have a cold or flu. On the upside, I performed well in yoga yesterday and in TKD last night. I feel lousy now, however. Whatever the cause, I look forward to *not* feeling this way, as it reminds me too much of how I felt during cancer treatment. I had bloodshot eyes yesterday; I don't look well either. This is confusing. Do I go to Dr. X or back to my general practitioner? Who's in charge now? I hope it just goes away on its own. This whole post-treatment recovery is like riding a yo-yo.

Super John's Helmet

In a couple of days I recover on my own from feeling down, no doctors required. My tiredness remains, but I am obsessing slightly less about it, even though I just mentioned it. But this fatigue is more like being sleepy than weak, and nowadays my body seems to be working like it's supposed to.

Tonight, taekwondo class is rigorous beyond reason, the way I like it. After some absurd combination of pushups and abdominal conditioning exercises and squats, all of which I complete, Super John approaches.

"Dave! You're looking good, bro! Fit!"

He pumps his fist at me in solidarity, for he's aware of my cancer and like a lot of other people in class, seems amazed that I'm not a decrepit shell of a man. Super John is a six-foot-three, 230-pound gregarious cowboy Tarzan, perhaps five years younger than me, and his compliment gives me an extra shot of energy. A natural athlete, he would fit neatly into an NFL starting lineup. He has taken to taekwondo with fluid ease. He has not been around the school as long as I have, though, and holds a lower belt ranking.

I would definitely hate to take on Super John in a street fight; it would not end well for me. However, in class I have a bit of an edge due to tenure, and a little thing I like to call "rules." Taekwondo is a sport with a specific set of rules, much like boxing. Sparring is controlled, and skill and experience can make up for a size disadvantage. Sometimes.

After conditioning we don sparring gear, and sure enough, Master Steel Curtain pairs me up with Super John. SJ is eager like a puppy, wanting to learn and progress. While the other students are being paired up, he leans over to me and says, "C'mon, Dave! Give 'er all you got! I want you to kick me in the head!"

"You want me to do what?"

"I gotta learn, Dave! Don't worry, I ain't gonna let you do it, but you gotta try!"

I look up. I doubt that I could kick Super John in the head if he stood perfectly still with his arms at his sides; the son of a bitch is five inches taller than me.

"Um, okay," I say, "I'll try."

He smiles and shakes my hand. "That's the spirit!"

Sparring commences and I throw a few kicks his way, tossing in some punches. Damn, it's hard to spar big guys; I feel like a little kid next to him. SJ nails me with a sidekick. After I recover my balance I note that that particular kick would be a career ender if I didn't have my chest gear on. He comes back again and I return the favor with a lovely sidekick to his gut. This stops him cold. He smiles like I just bought him a new deer rifle, and pulls out his mouthpiece.

"Good one, Dave! That's what I want! Now kick me in the head!"

"I'm trying!" I grunt, but I'm not sure he can understand me because I still have my mouthpiece in.

We start again and I notice that when he throws his right jab he dips his head, losing a few inches of altitude. When he does it again, I chuck up an outside-in crescent kick just outside his field of vision. BAM! I connect, spinning the foam helmet partially around his face.

Super John stops. I stop. I ponder the relative wisdom of my act while he straightens his helmet. Will he lose it now and kill me on the spot? He stares down at me, expressionless. I consider sprinting away.

"Yeah!" he yells, and begins laughing like a little kid. "That's what I'm talkin' about! *Whoo-ha!*" He shakes my hand profusely and can't stop grinning. You have to give the people what they want.

* * *

The oil puddle in the Corvette's garage bay continues to grow to alarming proportions. I step through the pain-in-the-ass process of putting a Vette on jack stands and climb under for an evaluation.

Oil pan gasket, I note, signifying a dismantling job sure to dwarf that of the Corvette's interior, requiring the position and patience of Michelangelo. Too much to bear, so I leave it for the night.

But sleep helps, and the next evening I'm back under the car. Multitudinous parts come off smoothly enough until I discover that the entire exhaust system must be removed, which is okay until I encounter the driver's side catalytic converter bracket. I *cannot* remove the rusty studs from the flange, even using Liquid Wrench, and break one stud off. I'm covered in grease and have to trash the laundry-room sink cleaning up so that I can imbibe more caffeine.

In a flash of despair and inspiration, I discover that a good old-fashioned hack saw will fit where I'm working, and I slice off the offending bracket. Perhaps this was the secret of the Sistine Chapel. *Up yours, bad Chevy engineer! And up yours, purists!* I finally get the pan off, halfway finishing the job. The Corvette has now officially gone from a symbol of Optimism to a pain in my ass.

9 THE COMEBACK

It's Friday night, May 16, and I'm at the dining-room table with Jenelle and the girls, enjoying a tasty Zinfandel and some fine food, which has thankfully regained its full taste after chemo. Carina is home from Rice for the summer and has taken to staying up late and sleeping ten hours a night like I would, if I could. I sleep anywhere from three to seven hours a night, and try to work in naps between my furious efforts to be normal—whatever that means.

It has been roughly two and a half months since my last radiation treatment, and the family has pretty well recovered from worrying about cancer. Well, *they* have.

We pass the salt and take turns describing our days (photocopy shenanigans at work, girl-fight on the bus, other typical human activities). I try to make the girls laugh (not that successfully) and they try to make Jenelle and me laugh (no problem). There is genuine mirth being served up with a side order of happy contentment. I decide to add to the high spirits of the evening by revealing an ingenious plan to affirm my newfound good health. I cannot wait to see how happy it will make Jenelle.

"Hey, by the way, I'm fighting in the tournament tomorrow."

In response Jenelle just stares at me, strangely quiet and impassive. She's doing a good job of reining in her enthusiasm, so I answer the obvious next question.

"Yeah, point sparring. Isn't that great?" I look at the girls and grin. "I'm so excited!"

"What?!" Jenelle thunders, a tone that seems a bit over the top for pleasant dinner conversation. "You're crazy! You're going to get hurt!"

"Nonsense!" I laugh with a dramatic wave of my good arm. "What could happen?"

She's looking at me as if I've just announced a new hobby of skyscraper diving or venomous snake juggling. "You're going to get hurt, is what could happen!" I'm getting an icy stare now. "Why would you do this?" She's apparently angry.

"What do you mean why?" I say, offended. "It'll be fun!"

The rest of the meal is not filled with mirth; I notice icicles forming on the water glasses. Jenelle really is angry with me, and I am resentful of her killjoy attitude. Why does she have to be afraid? Because she cares? Or maybe because she was there when her father died? Whatever. I refuse to cave in to her perfectly justified anxieties.

* * *

At our taekwondo school, being a black belt comes with various responsibilities, including helping out as a referee at a couple tournaments per year. So I ref all day until my own fight.

The tournament progresses from little kids on up through the age groups. Kaily fights and wins her Olympic-style match—she's a natural just like Carina was before she quit to go off to Rice. I am a proud papa.

At 3:00 the eighteen-year-olds finish and the announcer makes the call: "Next up: Open Black-belt Division." This is where the bad-asses reign, spanning ages nineteen to thirty-four. This will be followed by my group, the "Senior" division, for ages thirty-five to forty-four. I am forty-four – almost ready to be put out to pasture.

I put on my uniform and arrive at staging, ready to rumble, but look around and see slim pickings in the senior-citizen department. As it turns out, they don't have enough old guys today. This is probably because most older guys have enough sense to avoid this kind of thing. In fact, B.C., I myself wasn't too hot on the idea of getting out in the ring with all those fists and feet of fury. But now I find this dearth of gray unacceptable as I expect to make my big comeback. I damn well need to fight to show that I'm manly, tough, and most of all, recovered.

This is a conspiracy. Jenelle has kidnapped and locked away all the old guys so that I'll have to take it easy and not exert myself. I am not sure how she pulled this off, but I will not stand for it. I have things to prove.

I stomp down the risers and talk to the guy who stages the fighters. He thinks over the situation a moment and offers three choices: "Choice one," he says, looking me over. "Take a 'bye and go home with a trophy. And uninjured."

"Unacceptable. What else you got?"

"Choice two: I've got Master Todd over there." I look up the stands at Master Todd, a 245-pound Open Division thirty-something master instructor larger than Super John. Master Todd owns his own taekwondo school.

"Uhm. What else you got?"

"Choice three: Fight in your weight class, but in Open Division."

I remind myself that Open Division is where the bad-asses reside. "Who you got?"

"There happens to be a bracket of three guys, nineteen, nineteen, and twenty. They're all welterweights like you." He points them out. I even know one of them, Joe; he goes to my school. I ponder fighting Joe. He's a second-degree bad-ass (who will later go on to become a Marine badass), who has been in taekwondo since he was a little kid. Hmmm.

Four people make a proper bracket, which gives everybody the chance to fight twice (the losers fight for third place), so it appears that the stars have aligned for me and for this matchup. Technically, this is a proper shift. By AAU rules, a Senior can fight down in age to Open division, even if it's not the wisest thing to do.

I look the young guys over one more time. "Hell yes," I say, "I'll be the fourth! Let's go!"

The staging guy fixes my paperwork. We all put on our red foam hand and feet pads, and go down to the floor to wait for a ring to open up. I stand by the other three fighters and we nod, shake each other's hands.

"Hey, I just thought of something funny," I say. "I'm older than any two of you put together! Ha, ha!"

They exchange glances implying pity for my deteriorating mental condition. Joe smiles like I would smile at a nice old man on a park bench, then turns his attention to another fight getting underway. One of the guys in our group begins to stretch in ways that I would expect only from a rubber girl gymnast. I name him Gumby.

The ring opens up. I get paired off with Gumby and immediately feel pity for him, as in *I pity the flexible fool who fight me!* But I don't voice the sentiment. Gumby does not know what he is in for, because I have no fear: I have just survived chemotherapy and radiation, and I live everyday with the shadowy threat of Lumpy and his ilk. What is a boneless child fighter to me? I pity the fool!

Basically, I am out to kick Gumby's ass (but not literally, as the ass is not a scoring region). I am not out to injure the poor kid, but will damn well go for the win via points. The big-screen preview for this fight rolls before my eyes: the superannuated, formerly toxic Rocky overcomes awesome odds to claim his Big Comeback. The crowd goes nuts, Jenelle admits I was right, and young women weep with admiration as middle-aged men flock to taekwondo schools....

I fasten my helmet and pop in my mouthpiece. The center ref bows us in and lines us up, holding his arm out between us. He checks with the corner refs and the scorekeeper. They all give the nod. The ref yells *sejak* – "begin" in Korean – sweeps his hands together, and backs out of the way.

We go at it. A lot of taekwondo fighters like to first see what the other opponent does and then react with a counter move. I charge in like a bull on crystal meth. Take this, Lumpy! Bam! Whap! Gumby gets some good shots in, but so do I, and about a minute and a half in, I go ahead by one point. But that flexible son of a bitch is fast!

Gumby barely misses a couple of kicks, going *over* my head. None of my high kicks go over his head, or even land (after all, his reflexes are less than half as old as mine). I remain in fearless cancer-annihilation mode and charge in on him yet again, at which point he jams the crap out of me with a hard side kick, right under my left pec muscle—the radiation side.

There is no chest gear in point sparring, and it is a hell of a shot. I think: *Ooh! I'll feel that one in the morning!* But the refs fail to see it, or decide to pamper me by not scoring it, so we fight on without interruption. I nail him with a punch to the chest. Gumby stumbles backward and falls out of the ring, knocking over his coach's chair. He lands gracelessly on the wooden floor of the arena. *Whoa*, I think. *That was cool!*

I hear cheers and look up into the crowd. Mine is one of the last fights of the day, and the rest of the fighters from our respective schools and families are all there. I see the girls, and also Jenelle! That's right, she came after all, and is screaming wildly for me!

"Go David!"

"Go Daddy!"

"Go Mr. Baskett!"

Everybody is jumping up and down. I am loved and refreshed and invincible! Oh yes, all is well with the universe, and my marriage, and I am living life, by God, well past the speed of light—Warp Factor 9, at least. A fight like this, even for points, is primal, and in the thick of it there are no thoughts coming or going other than *survival*. My comeback is going better than I ever could have imagined. F_ _ _ cancer!

The center ref lines us up to start again. He lowers his hand between us. At this point I curiously choose to commit a strategic error: I abandon the Zenlike flow that got me this far, and instead become fixated on what kicks Gumby *might* throw, and what strategies I might then employ to counter these possible kicks. Because I want this to be the best comeback in history! I want to spin Gumby's helmet around his face with my foot. The center ref raises his arm and yells *sejak*.

As it turns out, aggressively punching an experienced nineteen-year old fighter in the chest is tantamount to flicking a tiger in the nuts. It is at this moment that Gumby, perhaps offended by the spectacle of being knocked over his coach's chair, launches into a spinning back hook kick, exactly as high as my head.

Due to my strategizing and the post-treatment attention span of a gnat, I can only stare at the beauty of his kick, as it seems to occur in slow motion. I have just enough time to think, *Whoa! That's a spinning back hook ki...* BAM! Gumby's heel tags me squarely on the bridge of the nose; the crack can clearly be heard on Carina's video. I stagger back, literally on my heels, as if I just took a punch from Mike Tyson. It is a YouTube moment.

After I finish staggering backward, I lean forward and grasp my knees. *Oh, yeah, this one's gonna bleed.* For a couple seconds, I'm fine; then comes the gusher. I spew blood on the mat and my gloves and all over the freaking place. Then comes the pain. I take a knee.

Somebody throws me a towel and I wipe some blood off myself and the floor. I manage to sit back on the coach's chair. Super John hops the rail from the stands. "Hey Dave, you all right?"

I am far from all right—holy shit, this hurts! But I say, "Yeah, feelin' pretty good, John. How do I look?"

I drop the towel and realize that I still have my gloves on, but cannot take them off because blood continues to pour out of both nostrils, and I am trying to catch it all in my hands. SJ looks closely at my face.

"Man!" he says, "that was the coolest thing I've ever seen! Mind if I get a picture?"

"What?"

He whips out a small digital camera and takes several pictures of my nose from various angles, your basic glamour close-ups.

A medic runs over, and without regard to how much additional pain it will cause, shoves what appears to be a pair of unlit cigarettes well up into my nostrils. He hands me another towel and I try to wipe up some more. I'm nothing if not neat when I bleed profusely in public.

It is at this moment that the center ref walks over. "Fighter!" he yells. "Do you want to continue?"

I'm now holding the towel up to my nose and leaning my head back. *Do I want to continue?* I think. *What about my comeback?* But with pain comes clarity: Gumby is not Lumpy. Gumby is Gumby, and he's strong and fast. The thought of another blow to the nose doesn't appeal to me at this juncture.

"Umm... no thanks," I say, sounding like a guy with a pair of unlit cigarettes up his nose. "I'll just go ahead and concede."

Suddenly a terrifying thought occurs—not that cancer has won, something much more immediate: *Jenelle is going to kill me!* She will finish the job Gumby so convincingly began. I replay in vivid detail Jenelle's speech about how she had not wanted me to fight, knowing how this thing would end in that psychic way of a wife— although she did not spoil the surprise by forecasting what kind of kick Gumby would throw. It can really piss her off when I ignore her and she's right.

My nose swells up to the size of half an avocado; I receive a bag of ice. Ice, however, is not the soothing balm for which I had hoped—now my face hurts like hell, and is also freezing cold. I continue to wait for the final fights to end with my head tilted back. I position myself behind other people so that a certain spouse cannot see me.

Super John disappears back into the stands and I hope that yet more fights will go on so that I won't have to face Jenelle, but soon the competition ends. I feel slightly vindicated that Gumby has taken second place.

* * *

I will have to ride home with Jenelle, as I cannot drive with my head tilted back and an icepack covering half my face. But I don't want to get beat up a second time in one day, even if the weapon is just an *I told you so.*

Jenelle and the girls run down from the stands. I must look pitiful; Jenelle appears to feel sorry for me.

"Are you mad?" I ask.

She just shakes her head, baffled, as if to say, *Men!*

Neither daughter is too concerned with the swollen bits or ice packs, as both were competitive gymnasts for years; we still have a reserved parking spot at our favorite orthopedic sports clinic. Carina shows me the kick on videotape, and Kaily seems to think it was pretty cool.

Because Jenelle is at least pretending not to be mad, I am happy, ecstatic even. Pain and damage aside, or perhaps even because of the pain and damage, that fight was cool! Because I am alive! I have lived! Sure, I took last place and got the crap beat out of me, but I have really lived! F_ _ _ cancer!

Back to School

About a day and fifty blood loogies later, I realize that the powerful side-kick to my chest has cracked a rib. I come to this conclusion because it hurts like a Sioux warrior's arrow whenever I bend over, cough, lay down, get up, laugh, or breathe deeply. My nose, meanwhile, is none too happy to have been sacrificed in the name of living life to its fullest, and the bruises around it turn green.

I wait one more week, then return to taekwondo class. As I open the door to the *dojang,* I brace myself for the walk of shame. I will be looked down upon as a weak loser by all of my fellow students. I bow in, and step out onto the mat.

Instead, I am The Man. Children and adults rush to gather 'round and look at my nose. Teenagers view me with awe. I am a rock star! Fellow old guys surround me, obviously wishing they too had cracked a rib and broken a nose, but *they* didn't have the nerve to stand up to their wives. Pansies! Who's The Man? Who just *lived*? Cancer boy, that's who! F_ _ _ cancer!

We condition like hell, put on our gear, and spar. I get paired with one of the high-end super-athletes, home from Harvard. Sparring with these elite, nationally competitive young guys is always a pleasure. He takes it easy on me and I have more fun and live some more. Next I get paired off with a colored-belt old guy (my age). We are having a casual session and I'm not paying too much attention. He chucks up a side kick, landing directly beneath my left pec muscle. The pain takes my breath away even though I have chest gear on. I stop sparring on the spot and take a knee. I'm done for the evening, maybe the year. Perhaps I should have waited. I don't feel like The Man anymore. Some comeback this has turned out to be.

* * *

I retreat to the garage to lick my wounds and find Vette-shaped distraction. I have ordered new weatherstripping online and it awaits me in an oversized cardboard box. Hours of hyper-caffeinated scraping later, the new pieces are installed with lots of gooey black adhesive. I leave the car's top off and the doors open while the glue dries.

The next evening it's time to check my handiwork. I have to put a lot more muscle into screwing the targa top in place than I would have guessed—it's more like a wrestling match—but finally it's done. The weatherstripping looks good; professional. Oh yes, I am the greatest Corvette handyman ever. But now the doors won't close when the windows are up. *That's odd.* A trip online reveals that I must pull off the door panels and adjust the windows to account for the fresh rubber.

Adjusting Corvette windows is not the intuitive process I had anticipated. After an hour of loosening and tightening bolts, sweating and sliding glass around in random directions, the doors now close. I reinstall the door panels; things are looking up. I pull out into the driveway and whip out the garden hose to check for leaks.

I'm not sure how this is possible, but it appears that more water pours into my car with the windows closed than it would if they were open. Deep pools have formed on my new seat covers. Without bothering to pull back into the garage, I yank both door panels back off. It is at this time that the neighbor boys decide to play basketball. I wave and say hi, but they only stare, perhaps because the sun is beating down on me and I'm sweating more than ever, or perhaps because my shorts are all wet from sitting in the Vette's seats. Their game seems to pause whenever I cuss at bolts or pieces of rubber.

Both windows have now been further adjusted. However, only one door will close when its window is up; the other looks like it might never close again. I pull back into the garage for the night. I hop out and find three oil spots on the driveway, right under where the freshly repaired oil pan was.

So I've officially and inextricably re-entered Corvette hell. For whatever reason, I thought it would be different this time. If the Vette were a horse I'd put it out of its misery. The car taunts me; it is a monster; it is Lumpy incarnate on wheels.

10 THE NEW

One of my new life philosophies is that there are diamonds hiding in the piles of shit that life dumps along the primrose path. For example: Gumby's hook kick has straightened my nose slightly. I'm still looking for the diamonds in my Vette-shaped pile of shit.

June 3

Journal Entry:

I did not work on the Corvette yesterday.

I thought this Vette would be better. But it's turned out to be the same old thing in a different color. Each repair and the optimism it generated has been followed by an even worse period of defeat and despair. The struggle to fix the Corvette feels like a continuation of my battle with Lumpy, and that leads to the suspicion that I'm stuck in fighting mode and can't snap out of it. Is this new insight my diamond or just a sign that I should post the car for sale on Craig's list? Maybe both. I think I should quit fighting now. I *will* quit fighting now.

* * *

It is June fifth. My ribs have mostly stopped hurting and my nose, though still tender, has no more traces of bruising. My sense of well-being continues to heal as well. It begins to sink in that I have time left—years, I hope; decades would be nice. I have three months between PET scans and the next one won't happen until July, which means that right now I have one more month where I don't have to worry about a damn thing. I am allowed to feel cancer-free—there is nothing to repair.

Another week passes, and the serenity sticks. Mostly. I still have aftershocks of anxiety now and then.

Running

I have disliked, or more accurately, *hated* running for decades. I have found it to be a chore and a pain, and when people look at me and say, "Hey, you look pretty fit. Do you run?" I answer by saying "Only if somebody's chasing me." But that seems so B.C. now.

I want to kill the aftershocks of anxiety, and decide that there is only one logical course of action: more exercise! I look out across the golf course and think about how fun it might be to run down some of those man-made hills before the golfers show up in the morning in their plaid shorts, gimme-visors, and expense-account bellies.

Journal Entry:

I jogged yesterday. I went out on the golf course. It is cushioned and full of hills. It didn't take long to feel out of breath.

I begin to run and run often, and quickly make a discovery: post-cancer running is fun; it is a narcotic. Not only is it exercise, which is already an opiate, but I get a smooth rush of endorphins afterward. It's the best of both worlds.

Weeks pass and it feels yet again like all my spare time is gone, even though I haven't repaired the Corvette lately. Where is my time going? I add up this week's workouts on my fingers. That's two taekwondo classes, three weight training sessions, two yoga classes, and three runs. I'm out of fingers. *Whoa,* I think, *that's fairly extreme, even by my own standards.* That's way more than I exercised B.C. Perhaps I'm still a little scared of Lumpy's ghost.

I don't want to go over the top; I merely want enough exercise to prevent a Lumpy comeback, keep me strong in case I have to go back for more treatment, take the edge off of my anxieties and keep me sane. Maybe eight sessions a week is more reasonable.

June 17: Six-Month Cancer Anniversary

Journal Entry:

I've been treating myself well, writing, sleeping well, taking naps, and I jogged. I've been to yoga every Monday and Friday, went to TKD last night, and generally things are going physically in the right direction.

Note that I said "physically in the right direction," as opposed to mentally, which seems to be a different story entirely. Mentally, I feel like Ebenezer Scrooge the morning after. I am in a mad rush to make up for lost time, to work toward a better life. I am locked and loaded and ready to devour this earth and every experience it has to offer that won't land me in jail. Six months since diagnosis? It feels like six years. Or six days. It feels like I've been marooned on an island where someone tried to kill me, but I killed him instead. And now time has been compressed and expanded all at once.

I know that I will lose eventually. At some point I will no longer be able to feel strong and vital, to sweat and push. I will become weak and frail and sore, unable to run as fast or kick as high. I will run more slowly and then walk and then shuffle and then wheel myself, and then I will stop. I do not know the schedule for that descent; it could be six months or thirty years.

But because it could be six months, I drink a cocktail of euphoria, fear, desperation, joy, and thankfulness each time I complete a yoga class or spar or a run on the golf course. It is my way of giving back. I am saying to God, "Look at me! I use the body that you have given me and push it to its limits while I can! Thank you for allowing me to do this today."

That comes off sounding a bit spiritual. B.C. I was as spiritual as a plastic water bottle or Bic pen; I was going to be spiritual *later*. But for me, the cliché works: There are no atheists in fox holes.

Knowing What I Know Now

During this whole ordeal, I wished hard and prayed and hoped and envisioned. And things came to pass, but not those things I planned, nor how I planned them. I found signs in every little event, relevant or not. Knowing what I know now, I would have exercised just as much, but might have waited a little longer for my comeback fight (I might still be waiting for that one). I tended to get ahead of myself and rushed to feel "normal." Knowing what I know now, I'd pace it better and cut myself some slack. I worried a lot when ambiguous news came; now I understand that cancer news, like the daily news of life itself, is seldom black and white.

What else? I would not have bought that Corvette. I would have broken the initial cancer news to Kaily more gently. I discovered that battles with Lumpy, that son of a bitch, could be won decisively. That's one of the most important lessons of all: cancer does not necessarily equal death; it can mean life, even a better life, whether it's a short one or a long one. I would not change my ability to feel more deeply serene, and would not give back my newfound spirituality or connection to those who have gone before me.

Spirits

Early morning cool is a relative term in a Texas June. I walk through the gate of the golf course just before sunrise, my shirt already off. I run the man-made meadows and bulldozer-wrought dunes. A single white crane stands by the foggy creek, and the scene looks like a Japanese painting. The crane takes wing as I approach.

I have discovered by happenstance that the combination of nature and running allows a spiritual connection, quite similar to the one I felt while bolted down to The Beast.

I don't run just for me, either. I run for the spirits of others, especially cancer patients. I run across a tee box and it feels like souls are hovering around me, waiting for something. *What do you want?* I think. *An invitation?* For some reason this feels like the right answer, so I go ahead and invite them on board—the dead and the dying, the old and the young. Anyone who has or had cancer gets to sit on my shoulders, except for the kids who get to sit up top. I feel them begin to climb on, inside me. But still, what do they want with me? Well, what would I want if I were some dead guy? To feel the wind rush in and out the lungs of the living; to feel the burn, the long strides, the sweat. What it feels like to have a strong body.

The presence of these spirits is not merely symbolic, nor is it a desperate stretch for a metaphor. It is very real to me. Running out here allows ghosts and souls to come inside; I feel them as they embrace my life force and experience the simple joy of physical exertion. They are a portal for me and I for them. They love the speed; they want to go faster! C'mon! Only a couple of hills left! I become consumed with their presence and realize that they were young and able once; they were strong, had lungs, could run like this, or at least dreamed of this.

Down a bank and the morning air flows past my sweaty skin, feeling almost cool. This must feel like ninety miles an hour to a dead person. The meaning of this morning becomes clear: Days on Earth are not all about pain and stress, or fighting off sickness and death, but also about running free with strength and speed. More of the spirits climb aboard, but I don't find myself slowing with their weight. Instead they push me and I can run even faster. I run faster than I could by myself at the end of this long jog—a cancer patient living my silly life in the silly suburbs and running around a golf course.

At this moment I share with them what heaven is like on Earth and they lift me up and make me swift. All of us sprint full-speed over the top of the last hill, thrusting our arms into the air just like Rocky, dancing and screaming, "F _ _ _ cancer!"

And the neighbors stare.

Onward

If this story really was the "Rocky" of cancer, then this book would have ended right there at the top of the grassy hill. Or maybe it would end with me being carted off to the loony bin. But that's not the way it works. Time passes.

The reader, cancer patient or not, might like to be told that cancer, mortality, and the stresses of daily life no longer bother me, for I am a veteran cancer warrior who has found full-time serenity. Myth buster: close, but not quite.

Post-treatment life has its own tidal flows. There are highs and mellow, placid stretches that go for weeks on end, but there are also ebbs. With each PET scan or follow-up exam, I drop back into the muck of anxiety and fear. Waiting for results does not get easier as I had thought it would; in fact, it becomes more difficult, perhaps because I feel that I have more to lose now: more good health and quality of life, more of the world I didn't use to notice. The next time I walk into Dr. X's office for results, I can damn well guarantee that I will feel fear that Lumpy's father has been found. And so it goes, like Russian roulette.

My follow-up PET scans have been clear so far. After the results the tide rises again and finds me buoyant. Life has become joyous by letting go; it's full of satisfying little moments and empathy for the people in our club and people in general (a much larger club). Every once in a while, though, I'll stop and probe Lumpy's old residence, now occupied by scar tissue. Will he return? Are these lymph nodes in my throat slightly soft, or hard and enlarged like a frozen blueberry? They seem okay, but still.... For me, the background fear never fully goes away, always playing like Fox News in waiting rooms, incessant and unsettling. Like I did with the televisions, I can try to ignore this fear. I also like to overwhelm it with feelings of pleasure in watching sunrises and sunsets, sharing laughter, acting crazy, participating in life and having new experiences. And I still try to crush the fear through exercise, but I cannot run fast enough or kick hard enough to escape the demon named Lumpy. I have been affected; damaged.

So because there is no other choice I learn little by little to share my lagoon with this shark, and I live life how it was meant to be lived *because* he is there. And it is a good life, better in many ways than the one before.

But in the still moments I sometimes wonder: when will the shark turn? And when he's not looking, I flip him off.

TOP 10 ENTRY-LEVEL CANCER RULES

10.   You will die, you just don't know when.

9. Probings are like living near a train—after a while you won't even notice.

8. Learn to enjoy watching needles penetrate your flesh.

7. Memorize this two-part mantra: "Drivin' the car? Drivin' the car."

6. Chemo and radiation give the hangover that keeps on giving.

5. Fear and Anxiety prefer to visit at 3:00 AM and stay for hours.

4. If the need to feel that death is imminent occurs, Google your diagnosis.

3. There will be tiredness on a biblical scale.

2. Damaging rays will bombard you from an insidious device; this is called TV news.

1. Don't give up! Fight! F_ _ _ cancer!

ABOUT THE AUTHOR

As of September, 2014, David Baskett, author of *The Opposite of Chaos,* and a forthcoming darkly-comic, horror/thriller, is alive, fifty, travelling, writing and exercising. And getting probed and scanned (much less frequently), just in case Lumpy's father decides to make a showing.

So far, so good....